Childhood Emotional Abuse: Mediating and Moderating Processes Affecting Long-Term Impact

Childhood Emotional Abuse: Mediating and Moderating Processes Affecting Long-Term Impact has been co-published simultaneously as *Journal of Emotional Abuse*, Volume 7, Number 2 2007.

Childhood Emotional Abuse: Mediating and Moderating Processes Affecting Long-Term Impact

Margaret O'Dougherty Wright, PhD
Editor

Childhood Emotional Abuse: Mediating and Moderating Processes Afecting Long-Term Impact has been co-published simultaneously as *Journal of Emotional Abuse,* Volume 7, Number 2 2007.

Routledge
Taylor & Francis Group
New York London

First Published by
The Haworth Maltreatment & Trauma Press, 10 Alice Street, Binghamton, NY 13904-1580 USA

The Haworth Maltreatment & Trauma Press is an imprint of The Haworth Press, 10 Alice Street, Binghamton, NY 13904-1580 USA.

This edition published 2012 by Routledge

Routledge
Taylor & Francis Group
711 Third Avenue
New York, NY 10017

Routledge
Taylor & Francis Group
2 Park Square, Milton Park
Abingdon, Oxon OX14 4RN

Childhood Emotional Abuse: Mediating and Moderating Processes Affecting Long-Term Impact has been co-published simultaneously as *Journal of Emotional Abuse*, Volume 7, Number 2 2007.

Library of Congress Cataloging-in-Publication Data

Childhood emotional abuse : mediating and moderating processes affecting long-term impact / Margaret O'Dougherty Wright, editor.
p. cm.–(Journal of emotional abuse ; v. 7, no. 2)
Includes bibliographical references and index.
ISBN-13: 978-0-7890-3711-4 (hard cover : alk. paper)
ISBN-13: 978-0-7890-3712-1 (soft cover : alk. paper)
1. Psychological child abuse–Complications. I. O'Dougherty Wright, Margaret. II. Series.
[DNLM: 1. Child Abuse–psychology. 2. Stress Disorders, Post-Traumatic–therapy. 3. Adult Children–psychology. 4. Parent-Child Relations. 5. Rejection (Psychology) W1 JO638M v.7 no.2 2007 / WM 170 C5341 2007]
RC569.5.P75C45 2007
362.76–dc22 2007044292

I would like to dedicate this special volume to Dr. Norman Garmezy, my advisor, mentor, and dearest friend, for his vision in helping those who are vulnerable to become resilient.

ABOUT THE EDITOR

Margaret O'Dougherty Wright, PhD, is Associate Professor of Psychology at Miami University in Oxford, Ohio. She received her PhD in Clinical Psychology from the University of Minnesota and completed her clinical internship training at UCLA's Neuropsychiatric Institute. Her research interests focus on the long-term consequences of child maltreatment across the lifespan with particular interests in: (1) the interpersonal functioning of adult survivors of abuse in dating, couple, and parent-child relationships; (2) ways in which childhood abuse may be linked to further exposure to abuse and victimization, with a focus on maladaptive interpersonal schemas, risky behavioral choices, and substance use; (3) explorations of protective processes that may foster resilience and recovery in child abuse survivors, such as family relationships, social support, coping strategies, spirituality, and meaning making; and (4) ethical issues in training clinical psychologists to work effectively with victims of child maltreatment, including factors influencing compliance with mandated reporting and appropriate use of self-disclosure in work with trauma survivors. She has published numerous chapters on the topics of vulnerability and resilience, as well as empirical articles focused on recovery following traumatic experiences.

Childhood Emotional Abuse: Mediating and Moderating Processes Affecting Long-Term Impact

CONTENTS

About the Contributors

Jessica S. Benas, MA, is a graduate student in the Department of Psychology at Binghamton University. She received a BS in Human Development from Cornell University in 2002 and her MA from Binghamton University in 2006.

Aubrey A. Coates, MA, is currently a doctoral student in clinical psychology at Miami University. Her research and clinical interests include the impact of childhood maltreatment on children's psychological well being, in particular difficulties related to emotion regulation.

Emily Crawford, MA, is pursuing her doctorate in clinical psychology at Miami University in Oxford, Ohio. Her research interests focus on the prevention and education of violence against women, in particular, drug-facilitated sexual assault. She is also interested in sexual communication among college students, and the interpersonal consequences of childhood abuse experiences, including psychological maltreatment, and the factors that help promote resilience.

Sarah E. Crossett is a graduate student in the Department of Psychology at Binghamton University. She received a BS in Psychology from Western Michigan University in 2003.

David DiLillo, PhD, is Associate Professor and director of the Clinical Psychology Training Program at the University of Nebraska-Lincoln. He conducts research in the area of family violence and couple relations. He is particularly interested in the long-term impact of child maltreatment. Dr. DiLillo's work is funded in part by a NIMH grant exploring associations between childhood abuse history and adult marital and parent-child functioning.

Brandon E. Gibb, PhD, is Assistant Professor and Director of the Mood Disorders Institute in the Department of Psychology at Binghamton University. He received a BA in Psychology from the University of Georgia and a PhD in Clinical Psychology from Temple University. He completed his Predoctoral Internship at the Brown University Clinical Psychology Training Consortium. His research focuses on cognitive vulnerability-stress theories of depression among children and adults, with a particular emphasis on the development of cognitive vulnerability to depression.

Terri L. Messman-Moore, PhD, received her PhD from Oklahoma State University and is currently Associate Professor of clinical psychology at Miami University. Her research interests include the impact of childhood maltreatment and sexual violence on interpersonal functioning and health-risk behavior among young women.

Tamara L. Newton, PhD, is Associate Professor, Department of Psychological and Brain Sciences, University of Louisville, conducts research on stress, trauma, and their consequences for mental and physical health, particularly among women.

Andrea R. Perry, MA, is a doctoral candidate in the Clinical Psychology Training Program at the University of Nebraska-Lincoln. Her research and clinical interests include child maltreatment, adult romantic relationships, and processes that mediate these constructs.

James Peugh, PhD, is Assistant Research Professor at the University of Nebraska-Lincoln. He conducts research in the areas of multilevel structural equation modeling, missing data handling, and assumption violations in latent variable modeling.

Dorothy J. Uhrlass, MA, is a graduate student in the Department of Psychology at Binghamton University. She received a BA in American Studies from Fordham University in 2004 and her MA from Binghamton University in 2006

Rebecca A. Weigel, MA, is a clinical psychology doctoral student at the University of Louisville. Her research interests encompass posttraumatic stress disorder and emotion, gender differences in biobehavioral markers of stress and disease, along with women's health issues more broadly.

Tuppett M. Yates, PhD, is Assistant Professor in the Department of Psychology at the University of California, Riverside. She is a graduate of the University of Minnesota's Joint Doctoral Training Program in Developmental Psychopathology and Clinical Science. Her research focuses on the developmental sequelae of childhood adversity with respect to both psychopathology and resilience.

INTRODUCTION

The Long-Term Impact of Emotional Abuse in Childhood: Identifying Mediating and Moderating Processes

Margaret O'Dougherty Wright

Until recently there has been limited attention paid to the long-term consequences of childhood emotional abuse (also known as psychological abuse), in contrast to the significant attention paid to the long-term effects of childhood physical or sexual abuse (Barnett, Miller-Perrin, & Perrin, 2005; Binggeli, Hart, & Brassard, 2001). In part this has been because emotional abuse was not recognized as a distinct form of child maltreatment until quite recently, and there has been considerable difficulty defining and assessing emotional abuse. Unlike physical abuse,

Address correspondence to: Margaret O'Dougherty Wright, PhD, Department of Psychology, 100 Psychology Building, Miami University, Oxford, OH 45056 (E-mail: wrightmo@muohio.edu).

[Haworth co-indexing entry note]: "The Long-Term Impact of Emotional Abuse in Childhood: Identifying Mediating and Moderating Processes." Wright, Margaret O'Dougherty. Co-published simultaneously in *Journal of Emotional Abuse* (The Haworth Maltreatment & Trauma Press, an imprint of The Haworth Press, Inc.) Vol. 7, No. 2, 2007, pp. 1-8; and: *Childhood Emotional Abuse: Mediating and Moderating Processes Affecting Long-Term Impact* (ed: Margaret O'Dougherty Wright) The Haworth Maltreatment & Trauma Press, an imprint of The Haworth Press, Inc., 2007, pp. 1-8. Single or multiple copies of this article are available for a fee from The Haworth Document Delivery Service [1-800-HAWORTH, 9:00 a.m. - 5:00 p.m. (EST). E-mail address: docdelivery@haworthpress.com].

Available online at http://jea.haworthpress.com

doi:10.1300/J135v07n02_01

which results in immediate and observable harm, the immediate consequences of emotionally abusive behavior are more elusive. The actions and behaviors that comprise emotional abuse (humiliating, demeaning, threatening language or behavior, denial of affection, or isolating a child) are not uncommon occurrences in family life, and it has been difficult to determine the threshold for considering a particular act abusive. Many parents, if not most, have acknowledged criticizing, ignoring, or being unsupportive of their child on a given occasion (Barnett et al., 2005). So, in the emotional abuse area in particular, it has been hard to distinguish among less than adequate parenting, parenting mistakes, and emotionally abusive behavior. This has made it difficult for child protection workers, therapists, and other child-care providers to accurately assess if the emotional abuse involves a repeated pattern of parent-child interaction, or if the incident has been severe.

Yet despite these definitional and measurement difficulties, there is now considerable evidence that emotional abuse may be one of the most destructive and pervasive forms of abuse and that such abuse may also constitute a "core component" of all forms of child abuse and neglect (Barnett et al., 2005; Binggeli et al., 2001; Brassard, Germain, & Hart, 1987; Garbarino, Guttman, & Seeley, 1986). This realization has stimulated a great deal of research that has focused on documenting the long-term consequences of such abuse, which span intrapersonal, interpersonal, and intrafamilial domains. However, while there has been substantial research that has documented the link between emotional abuse and later negative adjustment, there has been far less research that has specifically addressed important mediators and moderators of this relationship. Research has rarely been driven by theory in this area and less attention has been given to the *processes* that lead to symptoms of distress or disturbed interpersonal functioning. The purpose of this special issue is to focus on empirical work emanating from a clear theoretical framework that examines these important risk-mediator-outcome relationships. For our understanding to be advanced in this area, it is critical that research begin to focus on *why* and *how* and *for whom* such abuse has such a pervasive impact across the life span. This work is critical in order to be able to identify points of intervention with survivors of emotional abuse. In this special issue we will present exciting new research that explores mediators and moderators of outcome for adult survivors of emotional abuse across biological, psychological, and social domains.

In the opening article of this special issue, Yates provides a comprehensive review of the empirical and theoretical literature examining possible neurodevelopmental consequences of childhood emotional abuse. She outlines a multi-level, integrated, transactional model for understanding how experience and biology might interact to eventuate in the specific maladaptive outcomes we have observed following childhood emotional abuse. Her review focuses on two mammalian stress response systems: the limbic-hypothalamic-pituitary-adrenal-meduallary (L-HPA) and the norepinephrine-sympathetic-adrenal-medullary (NE-SAM) systems. Yates explores evidence from animal and human studies that recurrent patterns of hostile, indifferent, degrading, and unpredictable emotional interactions between a caregiver and offspring can have negative and enduring effects on these developing stress response systems and that such alterations in stress responsivity contribute to the types of adaptational difficulties that have been identified in survivors of child psychological abuse, such as increased vulnerability to stress, anxiety, depression, and other problems of adaptation. Yates proposes that emotional abuse can be conceptualized as a type of chronic relational adversity and highlights the importance of studying how such abuse disrupts development across multiple domains, including social, emotional, self, cognitive, and biological processes. Although research in this area is in its infancy, the evidence that she reviews suggests that emotionally abusive experiences in childhood have the capacity to initiate persistent alterations in neurophysiological stress response systems that can derail development. Her review provides a much-needed integration of theory and research in developmental neuroscience for understanding childhood emotional abuse and its long-term consequences.

The next paper in this section by Newton and Weigel expands on our understanding of the potential biological consequences of interpersonal mistreatment. These authors explored whether a history of interpersonal mistreatment acted as a potential contributor to heightened cardiovascular reactivity during social interaction. Prior work in this area had indicated that elevations in blood pressure can occur following exposure to a close partner's hostile social interactions or actions that communicated disrespect or an attempt to dominate (Brown, Smith, & Benjamin, 1998; Ewart, Taylor, Kraemer, & Agras, 1991; Newton & Sanford, 2003). Newton and Weigel's study expanded on this prior work by examining patterns of cardiovascular reactivity in relation to a history of interpersonal mistreatment and explored the moderating effect of gender and ethnicity (African American and European American participants). The study utilized a mild interactive stressor–a brief, problem solving discussion with an opposite gender partner–to explore cardiovascular responses during actual dyadic interaction. Prior mistreatment was associated with higher resting blood pressure levels and heightened blood pressure reactivity, with some surprising gender and ethnicity patterns. Their research highlights the important role that exposure to chronic interpersonal stress may play in long term negative health outcomes, such as cardiovascular disease, and opens up exciting avenues for future exploration. This research project also provides an interesting laboratory analogue that might be very well suited to adaptation for children and their parents, and could provide an important window on early patterns of altered cardiovascular reactivity in children who have experienced parental emotional abuse.

The final four papers in this special issue focus more directly on identifying mediators and moderators of negative outcome in intrapersonal and interpersonal domains following childhood emotional abuse. The first paper by Gibb, Benas, Crossett, and Uhrlass provides an extension of prior work by Gibb and colleagues (Gibb, Abramson, & Alloy, 2004) linking a history of childhood emotional abuse by parents to a subsequent cognitive vulnerability to depression. This study examined the importance of the *source* of emotional mistreatment by including reports of parent emotional abuse as well as that of peer verbal abuse. Gibb and colleagues then tested a mediational model, which explored whether the victimization-later depressive symptomatology relationship was mediated by increased negative automatic thoughts and decreased positive automatic thoughts. The mediational model was fully supported, and victimization experiences were more closely related to heightened negative automatic thoughts rather than to diminished positive automatic thoughts. Interestingly, lower levels of positive thoughts were only related to emotional abuse by parents, not by peers, suggesting that the development of these thoughts may occur and be consolidated earlier and/or be more influenced by parental messages to the child. This was not the case for negative automatic thoughts, which were significantly associated with both peer and parental abuse. This paper raises a number of provocative questions that await further research study pertaining to the developmental antecedents of negative and positive automatic thoughts and suggests the need to study not only the source of victimization, but the timing of it as well, since such factors may lead to different developmental effects.

The papers by both Messman-Moore and Coates and Crawford and Wright illustrate the potential of attachment theory (Bowlby, 1982) and interpersonal schema theory (Benjamin, 1996; Young, Klosko, & Weishaar, 2003) to provide a useful framework for examining the deleterious consequences that can be associated with a history of childhood emotional abuse. Based on a broad base of empirical data obtained with normal and maltreated children, these theories propose that early interactions with caregivers, most notably parents, contribute to the development of cognitive schemas, or internal working models of self-in-relation to others (Baldwin, 1992; Bowlby, 1982; Cicchetti & Toth, 2000). These working models form templates for how the child expects to be treated by others based on how he or she was treated and whether the "self" is thought to be worthy of love, care, and respect. Exposure to experiences of emotional abuse in childhood is likely to threaten the security of these attachment relationships, and may result in maladaptive models of self (e.g., the self is flawed, defective, shameful, unlovable) and/or other (e.g., others are not trustworthy, they will not care for me, they may abandon or abuse me). If such schemas are persistent, they may interfere with the child's ability to form secure and satisfying relationships with others later in life.

To examine this possibility, Messman-Moore and Coates explored the relationship between childhood emotional abuse and later interpersonal conflict and examined whether schemas pertaining to mistrust, abandonment, deprivation, and defectiveness/shame mediated this relationship for women. Their measure of interpersonal conflict assessed difficulties across several different contexts (friendships, romantic relationships, work and school relationships). Difficulty in these areas was linked to emotionally abusive experiences in childhood, even after controlling for general parenting behaviors of warmth and control and this relationship was fully or partially mediated by three of the internalized schemas proposed. Messman-Moore and Coates also examined whether different ways of coping with these internalized schemas, through overly accommodating behavior, avoidant social behavior, or domineering and controlling behavior, mediated the particular schema of mistrust and abuse. Although all three coping styles were partial mediators of interpersonal conflict, domineering and controlling behavior was the most robust factor. This paper provided clear evidence that the long-term impact of emotional abuse may be perpetuated through the individual's internalization of this experience and provided rich evidence of the multiplicity of ways in which these childhood messages of abuse can shape self-perception and guide coping behavior.

Crawford and Wright's paper highlights the importance of considering the impact of multiple forms of abuse, neglect, and family dysfunction, since different types of child maltreatment frequently overlap. In addition, it hasn't always been clear in prior reports on the sequelae of emotional abuse whether observed findings are specific to the experience of emotional abuse or are the result of exposure to multiple abuse trauma. Their paper provides evidence that even after controlling for childhood physical abuse, sexual abuse, and problematic parental alcohol use, emotional abuse remains a significant predictor of both intimate partner victimization as well as self-reported acts of adult aggression. Crawford and Wright's study also explored whether specific early maladaptive schemas mediated the relationship between early emotional abuse and later relationship aggression experiences. Romantic relationships were selected as a focus of study because they were thought to be prime targets for the possible enactment of maladaptive "interpersonal scripts," given the demands for trust, intimacy, affection, and conflict resolution in such relationships. Two schemas, mistrust and emotional inhibition, emerged as full mediators of dating victimization and as partial mediators of perpetration of aggression, which paralleled findings reported by Messman-Moore and Coates with respect to interpersonal conflict. The schema of self-sacrifice also mediated dating abuse, suggesting that overly accommodating behaviors and compulsive caregiving may have been learned as a way of appeasing an abusive caregiver and thus coping with early abuse. Feelings of entitlement and insufficient self-control emerged as schemas that were uniquely associated with perpetration of aggression and not with victimization. These schemas suggested that some survivors may have learned patterns of interaction that reflected an identification with the abusive parent and indicated that issues pertaining to limited ability to tolerate frustration and a disregard for others feelings might lead to serious relational difficulty for some survivors.

The final paper by Perry, DiLillo, and Peugh provides an in-depth look at the impact that emotionally abusive and neglectful behavior experienced in childhood might have on later marital satisfaction and explored critical mediators and moderators of this relationship. This is a particularly important area of research and one in which there are very limited prior reports. Problems with trust, intimacy, closeness to others, and sexual difficulties have been identified as problem areas for abuse survivors in general (Davis, Petretic-Jackson, & Ting, 2001; DiLillo, 2001), and difficulties in these areas are likely to be very salient for adults who experienced contempt, ridicule, and rejection from their primary attachment figures. Perry and colleagues examined whether adult psychological distress played a mediating role in the relationship between emotional abuse and marital satisfaction. They also explored whether this mediational pattern was moderated by gender and remained significant even after controlling for exposure to all other forms of childhood abuse. Their findings revealed that symptoms of psychological distress were significant mediators of this relationship, and that gender did moderate this relationship, resulting in slightly different patterns for men and for women. For men, the symptom of paranoia was the strongest mediator. This finding is similar to the findings reported by Messman-Moore and Coates and Crawford and Wright for both men and women and suggests that schemas reflective of mistrust and suspiciousness of others are one part of the enduring legacy of childhood emotional abuse. For women, hostility emerged as most salient in interfering with marital satisfaction, suggesting a possible identification with the emotionally abusive parent and perhaps difficulty regulating one's temper and negative mood. The potential for bi-directional influences between psychological distress and marital difficulty is also discussed by the authors and represents an extremely important area needing further investigation.

The research presented in this special issue represents an important first step in moving beyond the need to document that emotionally abusive experiences in childhood are damaging to finding possible explanations for the persistence of these negative effects. The studies have also broadened the focus to a wider range of outcomes for both men and women and explored potential mediating and moderating mechanisms that were grounded in theory and that might hold potential promise as avenues for clinical intervention. It is hoped that this exploratory research will contribute to a richer understanding of some of the processes involved in carrying the effects of abuse forward to adult life, and most of all, will serve to inspire others to pursue research in this area.

REFERENCES

Baldwin, M. W. (1992). Relational schemas and the processing of social information. *Psychological Bulletin, 112,* 461-484.

Barnett, O., Miller-Perrin, C. L., & Perrin, R. D. (2005). *Family violence across the lifespan: An introduction* (2nd edition). Thousand Oaks, CA: Sage Publications.

Benjamin, L. S. (1996). *Interpersonal diagnosis and treatment of personality disorders* (2nd edition). New York: Guilford Press.

Binggeli, N. J., Hart, S. N., & Brassarad, M. R. (2001). *Psychological maltreatment of children: The APSAC study guides 4.* Thousand Oaks, CA: Sage Publications.

Bowlby, J. (1982). *Attachment and loss: Vol 1. Attachment* (2nd edition). New York: Basic Books.

Brassard, M. R., Germain, R., & Hart, S. N. (Eds.). (1987). *Psychological maltreatment of children and youth.* New York: Pergamon.

Brown, P. C., Smith, T. W., & Benjamin, L. S. (1998). Perceptions of spouse dominance predict blood pressure reactivity during marital interactions. *Annals of Behavioral Medicine, 20*, 286-293.

Cicchetti, D., & Toth, S. L. (2000). Developmental processes in maltreated children. In D. J. Hansen (Ed.), *Nebraska symposium on motivation: Child maltreatment* (Vol. 46, pp. 85-160). Lincoln, NE: University of Nebraska Press.

Davis, J. L., Petretic-Jackson, P. A., & Ting, L. (2001). Intimacy dysfunction and trauma symptomatology: Long-term correlates of different types of child abuse. *Journal of Traumatic Stress, 14*, 63-79.

DiLillo, D. (2001). Interpersonal functioning among women reporting a history of childhood sexual abuse: Empirical findings and methodological issues. *Clinical Psychology Review, 21*, 553-576.

Ewart, C. K., Taylor, C. B., Kraemer, H. C., & Agras, W. S. (1991). High blood pressure and marital discord: Not being nasty matters more than being nice. *Health Psychology, 10*, 155-163.

Garbarino, J., Guttman, E., & Seeley, J. (1986). *The psychologically battered child: Strategies for identification, assessment, and intervention.* San Francisco: Jossey-Bass.

Gibb, B. E., Abramson, L. Y., & Alloy, L. B. (2004). Emotional maltreatment by parents, verbal peer victimization, and cognitive vulnerability to depression. *Cognitive Therapy and Research, 28*, 1-12.

Newton, T. L., & Sanford, J. M. (2003). Conflict structure moderates associations between cardiovascular reactivity and negative marital interaction. *Health Psychology, 22*, 270-278.

Young, J. E., Klosko, J. S., & Weishaar, M. E. (2003). *Schema therapy: A practitioner's guide.* New York: Guilford Press.

doi:10.1300/J135v07n02_01

The Developmental Consequences of Child Emotional Abuse: A Neurodevelopmental Perspective

Tuppett M. Yates

SUMMARY. This article provides an empirical and theoretical foundation to support increased attention to neurodevelopmental processes in understanding the developmental sequelae of child emotional abuse (CEA). After reviewing the socioemotional consequences of CEA, an overview of the mammalian stress response system is provided, the deleterious impact of early psychosocial adversity on the organization and integration of this system is discussed, and the applicability of these findings for considering CEA and its developmental consequences within a multi-level, integrative, developmental psychopathology framework is explained. Building on evidence that CEA is likely to result in significant and enduring alterations in the neurobiology of stress response systems and, by extension, in neurodevelopment more broadly, specific suggestions for future research and practice are offered. This article encourages greater attention to CEA as a salient developmental experience

---

Address correspondence to: Tuppett M. Yates, PhD, University of California, Department of Psychology, 2320 Olmsted Hall, Riverside, CA 92521 (E-mail: Tuppett.Yates@ucr.edu).

The author would like to thank Amanda Tarullo and Margaret O'Dougherty Wright for their insightful comments on an earlier draft of this paper.

[Haworth co-indexing entry note]: "The Developmental Consequences of Child Emotional Abuse: A Neurodevelopmental Perspective." Yates, Tuppett M. Co-published simultaneously in *Journal of Emotional Abuse* (The Haworth Maltreatment & Trauma Press, an imprint of The Haworth Press, Inc.) Vol. 7, No. 2, 2007, pp. 9-34; and: *Childhood Emotional Abuse: Mediating and Moderating Processes Affecting Long-Term Impact* (ed: Margaret O'Dougherty Wright) The Haworth Maltreatment & Trauma Press, an imprint of The Haworth Press, Inc., 2007, pp. 9-34. Single or multiple copies of this article are available for a fee from The Haworth Document Delivery Service [1-800-HAWORTH, 9:00 a.m. - 5:00 p.m. (EST). E-mail address: docdelivery@haworthpress.com].

Available online at http://jea.haworthpress.com

doi:10.1300/J135v07n02_02

and to neurophysiological processes as a heretofore overlooked source of information about the relation between CEA and adaptation.
doi:10.1300/J135v07n02_02 *[Article copies available for a fee from The Haworth Document Delivery Service: 1-800-HAWORTH. E-mail address: <docdelivery@haworthpress.com> Website: <http://www.HaworthPress.com>*

KEYWORDS. Maltreatment, emotional abuse, L-HPA, NE-SAM, neurodevelopment, stress reactivity

INTRODUCTION

Since Kempe's landmark article on battered child syndrome in 1962 (Kempe, Silverman, Steele, Droegemueller, & Silver), child maltreatment has emerged from the shadows as a major public health epidemic (Margolin & Gordis, 2000). Despite a burgeoning literature on the developmental sequelae of child physical and sexual abuse, however, less attention has been directed to the study (and treatment) of child emotional abuse (CEA; Behl, Conyngham, & May, 2003). In reviewing the empirical and theoretical literature on CEA, this article calls attention to the relevance of developmental neuroscience for understanding CEA and its consequences across multiple levels of analysis.

With the entrée of special issues and forums dedicated to understanding CEA in the late 1980s and early 1990s (Cicchetti & Nurcombe, 1991; Garrison, 1987), and the founding of this journal in 1998 (Geffner & Rossman, 1998), CEA has become a legitimate area of empirical and theoretical inquiry. However, a lack of conceptual and operational clarity as to what constitutes CEA has hampered efforts to identify and ameliorate its detrimental effects (Cicchetti & Nurcombe, 1991; Iwaniec, 1995). In this paper, CEA includes behaviors alternately referred to as "emotional maltreatment/abuse," "psychological maltreatment/abuse," and "nonphysical harm," that describe a caregiving pattern that conveys to children "that they are worthless, flawed, unloved, unwanted, endangered, or of value only in meeting another's needs" (American Professional Society on the Abuse of Children [APSAC], 1995, p. 2). Although I discuss both hostile/controlling and neglectful/unresponsive caregiving behavior under the broad umbrella of CEA, different subtypes of CEA are likely to have different effects on development, though this hypothesis remains to be tested empirically.

The purpose of this paper is to present evidence of the impact of CEA on child development and adaptation with particular emphasis on putative neurophysiological processes that may inform our understanding of pathways toward and away from psychopathology in the aftermath of CEA. To this end, I begin by summarizing the psychosocial and behavioral consequences of CEA. I then review relevant data drawn from research on the neurobiological effects of childhood trauma to provide a venue for considering how experience and biology may transact to eventuate in specific maladaptive (or positive) developmental outcomes following CEA. Here, I focus on the mammalian stress response system, particularly the coordinated actions of the limbic-hypothalamic-pituitary-adrenal (L-HPA) and the norepinephrine-sympathetic-adrenal-medullary (NE-SAM) systems. I review evidence that adversity and caregiving quality influence the mammalian stress response system in ways that affect development and adaptation. I encourage the adoption of a theoretically informed, multiple-levels-of-analysis approach to future research and practice on CEA. Specifically, I argue that the integrative paradigm of developmental psychopathology provides a conceptual framework to orient future investigations and interventions. In conclusion, I discuss the empirical and clinical implications of a developmental psychopathology approach for future research and practice aimed at understanding and mitigating the deleterious consequences of CEA.

THE SOCIOEMOTIONAL CONSEQUENCES OF CEA

Prospective and retrospective investigations implicate CEA in the etiology of significant and enduring deviations in socioemotional development (see Hart, Binggeli, & Brassard, 1998 for review). In their longitudinal study of a high risk poverty sample, Egeland and colleagues demonstrated prospective relations between CEA and insecure attachment to caregivers, noncompliance, low persistence, low enthusiasm, poor concentration, and declines in cognitive and motor competence across the first several years of life (Egeland, Weinfield, Bosquet, & Cheng, 2000). By school age, CEA was associated with high levels of negativity, impulsivity, poor social competence, low academic achievement, and increased psychopathology (see Erickson, Egeland, & Pianta, 1989 for review). Among the first to recognize and document the negative effects of CEA, the seminal work of Egeland and colleagues has been followed by other studies that clearly demonstrate specific associations between CEA and negative outcomes (e.g., Herrenkohl, Herrenkohl,

Egolf, & Wu, 1991; Solomon & Serres, 1999). Retrospective research has extended these findings into adulthood, demonstrating associations between CEA and anxiety, depression, personality disorders, suicidality, low self-esteem, and health problems (Briere & Runtz, 1988; Johnson et al., 2001; Mullen, Martin, Anderson, Romans, & Herbison, 1996; Spertus, Yehuda, Wong, Halligan, & Seremetis, 2003). Moreover, in several studies, the negative effects of CEA have been equivalent to, or greater than, those following other kinds of abuse or trauma (Briere & Runtz, 1988; Claussen & Crittenden, 1991; Gross & Keller, 1992; Mullen et al., 1996; Spertus et al., 2003; Vissing, Straus, Gelles, & Harrop, 1991).

Clearly, CEA is associated with serious and negative emotional and behavioral consequences. Indeed, some have suggested that CEA is *the* core factor underlying the deleterious effects of child maltreatment broadly (Hart et al., 1998; Navarre, 1987). As is the case in the broader literature on child maltreatment (Cicchetti & Toth, 2000), however, extant research on CEA has focused on psychological and behavioral consequences and mechanisms of psychopathology to the relative exclusion of biological processes. This, despite the growing body of empirical research indicating that child maltreatment may influence neurodevelopmental processes to alter the structure, organization, and function of the brain and its neurobiological systems (De Bellis, Baum et al., 1999; De Bellis, Keshavan et al., 1999; De Bellis & Putnam, 1994; Glaser, 2000; Perry & Pollard, 1998). Efforts to understand the neurobiological and neurodevelopmental consequences of early adversity have yet to examine if and how CEA may shape developmental pathways at the level of physiology.

A NEURODEVELOPMENTAL PERSPECTIVE

Over the past 20 years, our understanding of the development and functioning of the mammalian brain has increased dramatically. The enduring capacity for plasticity at the level of form and function is a central feature of the brain with processes related to cell proliferation, migration, differentiation, and death enabling both recovery from injury and untoward deviations following adversity (Kolb, 1989). While many systems are affected by, and are integrally involved in, stress responsivity (see Bremner & Vermetten, 2001; Chrousos, 1998; De Bellis, Baum et al., 1999 for reviews), here I focus on the physiology and neurobiology of the core mammalian stress response systems that have been subject to the most empirical attention.

The Mammalian Stress Response

The mammalian stress response consists of two primary systems: the limbic-hypothalamic-pituitary-adrenal (L-HPA) axis regulates slower acting responses to stress and the norepinephrine-sympathetic-adrenal-medullary (NE-SAM) system underlies acute stress responses (Gunnar & Cheatham, 2003; Lopez, Akil, & Watson, 1999). In response to a perceived threat or stressor, the central nucleus of the amygdala activates the L-HPA and NE-SAM systems via connections with the hypothalamus and brainstem, respectively (Roozendal, Koolhaas, & Bohus, 1997). Operating at various sites throughout the central and peripheral nervous systems, these networks modulate behavioral, emotional, cognitive, metabolic, immunological, autonomic, and endocrine aspects of the mammalian stress response (Owens & Nemeroff, 1991).

The limbic-hypothalamic-pituitary-adrenal axis. The L-HPA axis, which consists of the hypothalamus, anterior pituitary gland, and adrenal cortices, regulates the longer acting and slower reacting stress response (see Figure 1; Vasquez, 1998). Following stress-induced amygdalar innervation, neurons in the paraventricular nucleus of the hypothalamus (PVN) secrete corticotropin-releasing hormone (CRH) into the hypophysial portal system that connects the hypothalamus to the pituitary gland. CRH travels through this system to the anterior pituitary where it stimulates the formation and release of adrenocorticotropic hormone (ACTH). Acting at receptors in the adrenal cortex, ACTH stimulates the release of glucocorticoids (cortisol in humans and primates, corticosterone in rodents) into the bloodstream. In turn, glucocorticoids act at receptors throughout the brain and body to suppress immune functioning, increase glucose conversion, reduce fear responses, influence learning and memory, reduce digestion, and inhibit further CRH secretion via negative feedback to the hypothalamus, pituitary gland, and hippocampus (Nelson & Carver, 1998).

The norepinephrine-sympathetic-adrenal-medullary system. In addition to its role stimulating the pituitary to release ACTH, CRH acts in the locus ceruleus (LC) of the brainstem to increase norepinephrine (NE) release and activate the sympathetic nervous system (SNS; see Figure 2; Valentino, Curtis, Page, Pavcovich, & Florin-Lechner, 1998). The NE-SAM system, which is comprised of the SNS and the adrenal medulla, stimulates

FIGURE 1. Schematic of the limbic-hypothalamic-pituitary-adrenal stress response system (L-HPA). In response to perceived threat or stress, corticotropin-releasing hormone (CRH) is secreted by the paraventricular nucleus of the hypothalamus. Acting in the anterior pituitary gland, CRH stimulates the production and release of adrenocorticotropic hormone (ACTH). ACTH acts in the adrenal cortices of the adrenal glands to stimulate the synthesis and release of glucocorticoids (i.e., cortisol in humans) into the bloodstream. In addition to its role of modulating long-term stress responses, cortisol provides inhibitory feedback to the brain (e.g., hypothalamus, pituitary gland, hippocampus) to modulate the subsequent production and release of CRH and ACTH. Connections among the hypothalamus and the amygdalar and hippocampal limbic structures are not shown here.

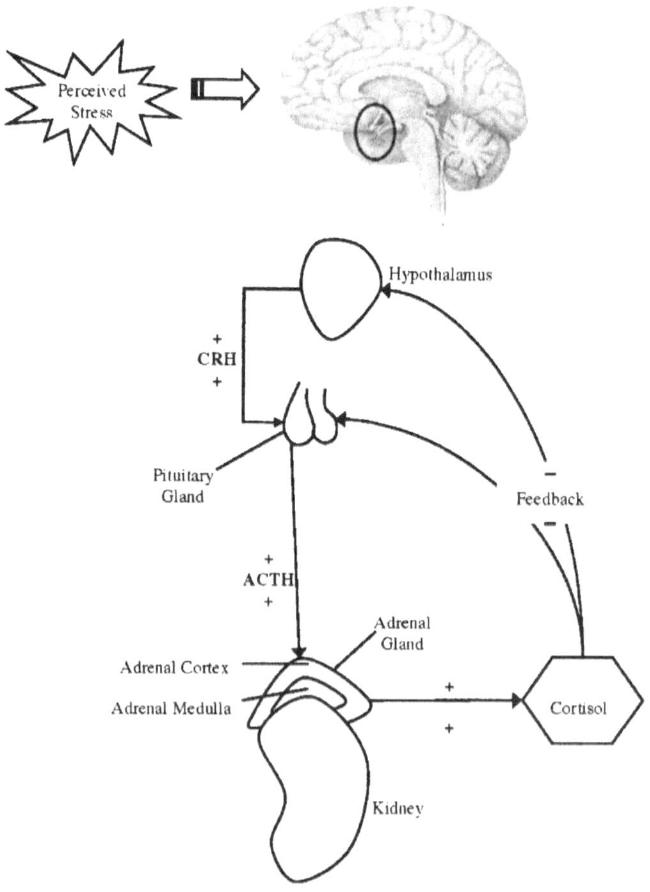

FIGURE 2. Schematic of the norepinephrine-sympathetic-adrenal-medullary system (NE-SAM). In response to perceived threat or stress, corticotropin-releasing hormone (CRH) is secreted by the paraventricular nucleus of the hypothalamus. Acting in the locus ceruleus, which is a nucleus in the brain stem, CRH stimulates the production and release of norepinephrine (NE). In turn, NE activates the sympathetic nervous system (SNS) and the release of acetylcholine (ACH) in the adrenal medulla of the adrenal glands. ACH stimulates the production and release of large amounts of epinephrine (E) and smaller amounts of NE into the blood stream to mediate acute stress responses. Connections among the hypothalamus and the amygdalar and hippocampal limbic structures are not shown here.

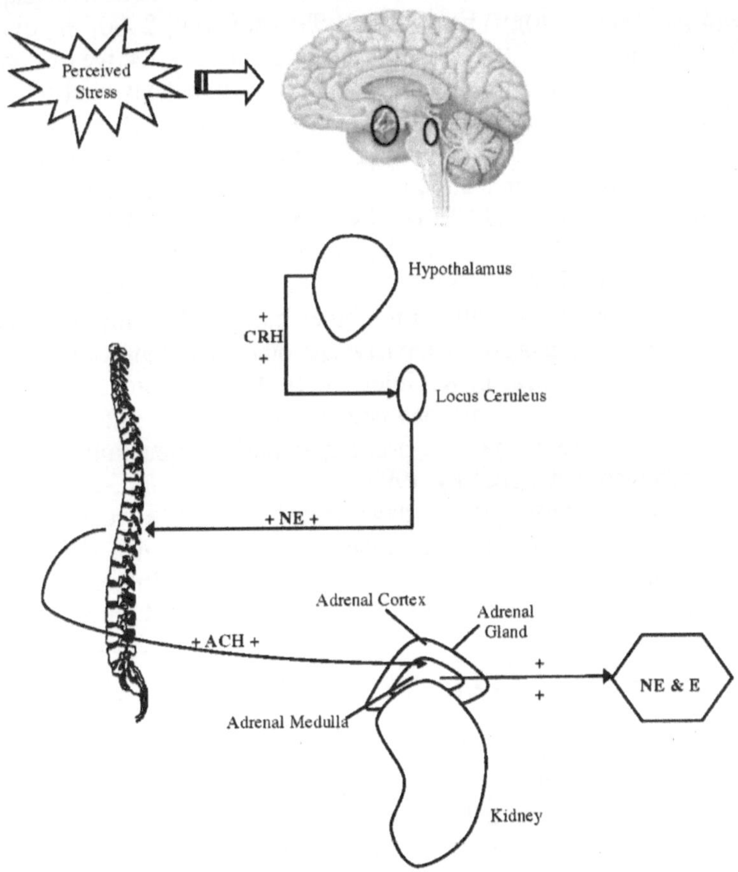

the production and release of NE and epinephrine (E) from the adrenal medulla into the blood stream where they act at receptors to elevate heart rate and blood pressure and ready the body for fight and flight responses to acute stressors (Koob, 1999). Together, the L-HPA and NE-SAM systems coordinate efficient and adaptive responses to stress via the peripheral release of adrenal steroids (i.e., glucocorticoids from the adrenal cortex) and catecholamines (i.e., NE and E from the adrenal medulla), respectively. Moreover, the coordinated action of these systems modulates processes related to neuronal migration, differentiation, synaptic proliferation, and, by extension, neurodevelopment (De Bellis, Keshavan et al., 1999).

Complementary coactivation. As primary stress mediators, glucocorticoids and catecholamines underlie pathways toward both positive adaptation and pathophysiology (Bremner, 1999; McEwen, 2000; Sapolsky, 1996). In the short-term, these systems are essential for effective responses to stressful stimuli, but dysregulation of these systems may contribute to enduring and pathological alterations as resources are directed away from long-term survival functioning in favor of short-term energy mobilization and response. Under normal circumstances, reciprocal connections within and between the L-HPA and NE-SAM systems serve to modulate the stress response (Nelson & Carver, 1998; Valentino et al., 1998). Simultaneous activation of the L-HPA and NE-SAM systems yields adaptive responding, but activation of one without the other may produce indiscriminate flight/fight reactions, depression, anxiety, and other symptoms of pathology (Yehuda, Southwick, Mason, & Giller, 1990). Furthermore, alteration of neurobiological stress systems may negatively influence other aspects of neurodevelopment (e.g., synaptic pruning, dendritic branching, neuronal death or endangerment; Sapolsky, 1996). Thus, alterations in L-HPA and/or NE-SAM stress response systems may mediate relations between early life stress and pathological outcomes (Bremner, Krystal, Sowthwick, & Charney, 1996; Cicchetti & Walker, 2003; Heim, Ehlert, & Hellhammer, 2000; Heim & Nemeroff, 2001; Kaufman, Plotsky, Nemeroff, & Charney, 2000).

PSYCHOSOCIAL ADVERSITY AND STRESS PHYSIOLOGY

Evidence from preclinical (i.e., animal) and clinical (i.e., human) studies converge on the assertion that adversity can instantiate neurophysiological alterations that undermine the adaptive organization and operation of mammalian stress response systems. Moreover, social factors, particularly the quality of early caregiving, have significant effects on the development, organization, and enduring efficacy of these systems. In this section, I review preclinical and clinical studies that point to probable neurodevelopmental effects of CEA and their implications for adaptive functioning.

Preclinical Studies

Animal research consistently indicates that adversity in early development has a negative impact on the organization and efficacy of neurobiological stress response systems (see Francis, Caldji, Champagne, Plotsky, & Meaney, 1999; Sanchez, Ladd, & Plotsky, 2001 for reviews). Moreover, studies suggest that the quality of the early caregiving environment is a major influence on observed relations between adversity and stress regulation (see Francis & Meaney, 1999; Levine, 2001 for reviews). Brief separations between rodent pups and dams in handling paradigms yield very different effects than maternal separation paradigms, which expose the pup to prolonged separation from the dam. Separated rats exhibit larger and longer glucocorticoid responses to stress, reduced glucocorticoid receptor density in the hippocampus and prefrontal cortex, increased CRH activity, and larger central NE responses to threat via the LC. In contrast, handled rats exhibit decreased CRH activity, increased glucocorticoid receptor density in the hippocampus, and generally reduced stress reactivity (Ladd, Owens, & Nemeroff, 1996; Plotsky & Meaney, 1993). In sum, a brief stressor (i.e., handling) appears to enhance neurophysiological stress modulation, while a prolonged stressor (i.e., separation) undermines it.

Interestingly, studies indicate that the quality of maternal care upon reunification is a key mechanism underlying these divergent responses to handling and separation paradigms. After brief handling, there is an increase in maternal grooming and arched-back nursing, whereas longer separations lead to disorganized caregiving behavior. Early handling alters maternal grooming and nursing behavior in ways that protect the structure and functioning of the rodent pup's stress response system, while extended separations undermine maternal caregiving in a way that compromises the development of the pup's stress response systems (Caldji, Diorio, & Meaney, 2000). Extending these findings to nonhuman primates, recent studies demonstrate that exposure to unpredictable resource availability in a variable foraging paradigm stresses Bonnet macaque monkey mothers, degrades the quality of caregiving to infant monkeys, and increases the offspring's stress reactivity (Coplan, Paunica, & Rosenblum, 2004). Additional studies have shown that normative individual differences in caregiving can influence stress response systems such that rodent mothers who groom and arched-back nurse their pups more tend to have more stress resistant offspring (Caldji et al., 1998; Liu et al., 1997). Finally, cross-fostering studies indicate that postnatal caregiving experience (e.g., taking a pup from a low grooming and arched-back nursing mother and cross-fostering it to a high grooming and arched-back nursing mother) modifies the pup's stress response systems, which demonstrates that these effects do not exclusively reflect genomic similarities (Francis, Diorio, Liu, & Meaney, 1999). These findings point to the importance of early caregiving quality for the development and operation of stress response systems.

Clinical Studies

Consistent with preclinical findings, clinical research indicates that early adversity may alter the neurobiology of stress response systems with enduring implications for human neurodevelopment and adaptation. Although the majority of research in this area has focused on populations exposed to traumatic stressors in childhood, growing evidence from broader samples supports preclinical findings that more subtle variations in the quality of early caregiving have salient effects on the organization of stress response systems. Together, these studies provide a strong evidentiary base for the assertion that CEA is likely to undermine the development and operation of human stress response systems with enduring negative implications for adaptation.

Research consistently demonstrates that child maltreatment contributes to marked deviations in normative neurobiological and neurodevelopmental processes related to the operation of the L-HPA and NE-SAM stress response systems. However, the specific direction of these effects (i.e., hypo versus hyperactivation) varies in ways that are not yet fully understood (see Cicchetti, 2003 for review). For example, in a large low-income sample of maltreated and nonmaltreated school-age children, Cicchetti and Rogosch (2001a) observed a pattern consistent with *hyper*cortisolemia among children with sexual or multiple abuse histories, but a pattern suggestive of *hypo*cortisolemia among physically abused children. Other researchers have suggested that initial patterns of hyperactivation may be followed by a progressive shift toward hypoactivation over time as a function of changing receptor densities (e.g., downregulation of glucocorticoid receptors in the anterior pituitary; De Bellis & Putnam, 1994). Despite changes as a function of maltreatment subtype, time elapsed since exposure, or other variables, it is important to recognize that both hypo and hyper stress reactivity have negative implications for development and adaptation (Heim et al., 2000).

While studies of abused children suggest that marked deviations in early caregiving contribute to pathological alterations in developing stress response systems, researchers have recently begun to study more subtle variations in parenting processes through the lens of developmental neuroscience (see Bugental, Olster, & Martorell, 2003 for discussion). For example, Gunnar and colleagues have shown that the quality of maternal care shapes the normative development of stress reactivity over the first year of life. Infants with responsive caregivers exhibit age-expected declines in L-HPA axis activity between 6 and 15 months of age, whereas infants with less-responsive caregivers display an atypical increase in cortisol reactivity between 6 and 15 months of age (Gunnar, Broderson, Krueger, & Rigatuso, 1996). Similarly, secure attachment relationships, which typically follow from a history of sensitive and responsive caregiving, are associated with more adaptive stress responsivity (e.g., lower cortisol elevations in response to a stressor) than insecure attachment relationships, which are associated with less responsive and consistent caregiving (Gunnar, Brodersen, Nachmias, Buss, & Rigatuso, 1996; Nachmias, Gunnar, Mangelsdorf, Parritz, & Buss, 1996). Particularly pronounced deviations in normative stress responses (e.g., marked elevations in stress-induced cortisol and heart rate) have been observed among children with disorganized attachment relationships, which typically follow from the kind of unsafe, unpredictable, or severely misattuned caregiving that may characterize CEA (Hertsgaard, Gunnar, Erickson, & Nachmias, 1995; Spangler & Grossman, 1993).

As observed in animal studies of cross-fostering, these effects are not mediated exclusively by genomic processes. Investigations of substitute care strongly suggest that observed relations between parenting quality and child stress responses transcend the contribution of genetic similarity. For example, in a study of 9-month-old infants, Gunnar and colleagues (1992) found that the child's response to a 30-minute separation from the caregiver was moderated by the quality of the substitute care provided (Gunnar, Larson, Hertsgaard, Harris, & Broderson, 1992). Infants did not evidence a stress response when placed with a responsive babysitter, but they did exhibit increased cortisol when placed with an insensitive babysitter. Similar findings have been observed in investigations of the relation between the quality of out-of-home child care and stress reactivity in young children, with high quality care setting associated with reduced levels of L-HPA dysregulation (e.g., Dettling, Parker, Lane, Sebanc, & Gunnar, 2000).

CHILD EMOTIONAL ABUSE AND NEURODEVELOPMENT

Preclinical and clinical research studies demonstrate that enduring alterations in the activity of the L-HPA and NE-SAM stress response systems may follow from adverse experiences in childhood. Evidence suggests that the quality of the early caregiving environment may moderate or mediate these relations. Moreover, even relatively subtle variations in the quality of early care appear to affect developing stress response systems. To date, however, few studies have examined whether these patterns generalize to CEA, whether effects differ across subtypes of CEA (e.g., unavailable versus intrusive care), and what the implications of these potential alterations may be for later development and adaptation.

The available literature suggests that recurrent patterns of hostile, indifferent, degrading, and unpredictable emotional exchanges in the caregiving milieu, as may typify instances of CEA, will have negative and enduring effects on emerging stress response systems and adaptation. Of the few studies that have included assessments of CEA in their investigations of stress responsivity, the majority indicate that CEA is associated with dysregulation of both the L-HPA and NE-SAM stress response systems. Bugental and colleagues (2003) found that young children who had been emotionally abused in the first year of life exhibited atypical elevations in basal levels of cortisol suggesting L-HPA axis dysregulation (Bugental, Martorell, & Barazza). A similar relation between CEA and elevated L-HPA axis activity has been found in a sample of adult children of Holocaust survivors who report a history of CEA (Yehuda, Halligan, & Grossman, 2001). With respect to noradrenergic functioning, Jones and colleagues (1997) found that intrusive parenting was associated with elevated catecholaminergic transmission suggesting hyperactivation of the NE-SAM system. In contrast to the studies reviewed thus far, Cicchetti and Rogosch (2001a) did not find differences in cortisol regulation patterns between children with a history of CEA and a high-risk nonmaltreated comparison sample. However, these authors note that the prevailing context of risk in this study may have overshadowed meaningful differences between children with and without histories of CEA.

In addition to CEA-induced alterations in stress responsivity, a growing body of evidence indicates that CEA may contribute to dysregulated stress response patterns indirectly. For example, CEA may moderate relations between physical or sexual abuse and stress-response alterations. In a study of depressed maltreated, depressed nonmaltreated, and nonmaltreated children, Kaufman and colleagues (1997) observed differences in L-HPA functioning following intravenous administration of CRH. As expected, depressed abused children evidence higher levels of ACTH release than both nonmaltreated groups; however, all the depressed maltreated children who exhibited increased ACTH release were living in homes with ongoing CEA.

In addition to direct effects on neurodevelopment via the introduction or mitigation of arousing stimuli, CEA may influence psychological processes that, in turn, affect the child's stress responsivity. Intrapsychic mechanisms, such as perceived control and predictability, can regulate the activity of stress response systems (Granger, Weisz, McCracken, Ikeda, & Douglas, 1996; Sapolsky, 1994). Thus, CEA may indirectly affect stress responsivity via representational processes (e.g., reductions in self-esteem; Gross & Keller, 1992) that might contribute to altered stress reactivity. As the mechanisms by which CEA undermines effective stress regulation come into focus, attention should shift toward the study of the adaptive consequences of CEA-induced alterations in stress physiology.

IMPLICATIONS FOR ADAPTATION

The specification of neurodevelopmental mechanisms in the pathophysiology of mental disorders is a prominent focus of contemporary experimental psychopathology (see Cicchetti & Walker, 2003 for review). Research suggests that alterations in the neurobiology of stress responsivity may contribute to contemporaneous and prospective adaptational difficulties that have been associated with CEA. Among school-aged children, for example, early adversity and consequent alterations in stress physiology have been associated with reduced social, cognitive, and emotional competence (Gunnar, Tout, deHaan, Pierce, & Stansbury, 1997; Hart, Gunnar, & Cicchetti, 1995). In adult samples, dysregulation of stress response systems has been associated with anxiety disorders and depression (Heim, Owen, Plotsky, & Nemeroff, 1997; Nemeroff, 2004). Available evidence suggests that CEA may cause deviations in normative stress response development that contribute to disorders of adaptation that have been associated with CEA.

In addition to the physiological consequences of CEA, recent findings suggest that there may be physiological causes of CEA. Animal research indicates that the intergenerational transmission of parenting behaviors may occur via experience-induced alterations in stress response physiology (Francis, Diorio et al., 1999). In an unpublished study by Martorell and Bugental (as summarized in Bugental, Martorell et al., 2003), parents who endorsed low levels of perceived power were more likely to show cortisol elevations in response to stressful interactions with their toddlers, which, in turn, contributed to punitive parenting. Thus, parents who respond to challenges in the caregiving relationship with physiological activation may be more likely to engage in punitive parenting practices. To the extent that CEA increases stress reactivity and decreases levels of self-esteem and self-efficacy, it may increase the probability of compromised parenting in the next generation. These findings support the assertion that, as a chronic relational adversity in childhood, CEA carries a high probability for inducing neurobiological deviations in development that are implicated in the pathophysiology of subsequent maladaptation, including the intergenerational transmission of child maltreatment.

A FRAMEWORK FOR FUTURE RESEARCH AND PRACTICE

In this paper, I encourage greater attention to putative neurodevelopmental processes that may be affected by CEA and that, in turn, influence social, emotional, and behavioral adaptation. To this end, I provide specific suggestions for future research and practice that incorporate psychobiological processes across multiple levels of analysis and intervention. As observed by Gottlieb and Halpern (2002), and as supported by the research reviewed here, the cause of development is neither biology, nor the environment, but rather the relation within and among developmental systems and their components. I contend that a multiple-levels-of-analysis approach to future research and practice is essential to our understanding of the specific relations within and among the psychosocial, behavioral, and biological systems involved in CEA and its developmental sequelae.

Directions for Future Research

Over the past decade, scholars have highlighted the need for interdisciplinary research efforts across multiple levels of analysis (Cacioppo & Berntson, 1992; Cicchetti & Blender, 2004). However, a relational view of causality in research requires more than information from multiple levels of analysis; it requires theoretically informed hypotheses that specifically consider relations across systems (Gottlieb & Halpern, 2002). Thus, interdisciplinary, multi-level research requires a conceptual framework that can accommodate multiple sources of information and appreciates that "there are psychological phenomena that derive from events at one level of analysis and that are only or more distinctly observable across levels of analysis" (Cacioppo & Berntson, 1992, p. 1023).

As an integrative conceptual framework that draws on the principles of core developmental theories and models, developmental psychopathology is especially well-suited for orienting future research and practice related to CEA within an interdisciplinary, multi-level systems approach (Cicchetti, 1993; Masten, 2006; Sroufe & Rutter, 1984). Developmental psychopathology localizes positive and pathological adaptation in the transactional relations between individuals and their internal and external environments, rather than as inherent to the individual or the environment (Cicchetti & Toth, 1997). This transactional view of development readily encourages the integration of biological and psychological levels of analysis within a common conceptual framework. Building on a developmental psychopathology framework and adopting multi-level paradigms, future research on the developmental consequences of CEA will advance us toward an integrative understanding of the neurophysiological and psychosocial transactions that follow from CEA to eventuate in particular adaptive outcomes. To this end, I offer the following suggestions for future research on CEA.

First, there is a need for greater clarity in defining CEA, and for improved measures to enable its reliable assessment across the developmental continuum (see Hart, Brassard, Binggeli, & Davidson, 2001 for a review of these issues). Similarly, given the tremendous value of experimental manipulations in animal research, there is a marked need for the development of animal paradigms that can approximate the human experiences of degradation, humiliation, and betrayal that typify much of child maltreatment, particularly CEA. Although there are significant limitations to the translation of findings across species, animal studies remain an important resource for initial hypothesis testing to inform clinical research and for identifying neurophysiological mechanisms of change that cannot be directly observed in human samples.

Second, just as the conceptualization and assessment of CEA will change across time and context, so, too, must future research trace patterns of adaptation and transaction over time. As discussed previously, the physiological and behavioral effects of CEA will vary as a function of the developmental status of the individual at the time of exposure and of the time that has elapsed since exposure (Nelson & Carver, 1998; Teicher, 2002). Similarly, there is a need for longitudinal research designs to test if and how CEA-induced physiological changes affect long-term adaptation. A longitudinal, process-level approach to the study of CEA and adaptation will permit the specification of causal relations, as well as the identification of intervening factors that may moderate pathways towards and away from pathological outcomes.

Third, future investigations must explicitly address the dynamic nature of development and adaptation as outgrowths of transactions among multiple, embedded, overlapping, and interacting systems. Specific features of CEA, including age of the child at time of onset, gender of the child victim, gender of the perpetrator, frequency of abuse, presence of other forms of abuse, and how the child perceives and makes meaning out of the abuse may influence the impact of CEA on the child's physiology, psychology, and adaptation (Cicchetti & Rogosch, 2001a; Manly, Kim, Rogosch, & Cicchetti, 2001; Mullen et al., 1996). Moreover, specific investigations must examine if and how hostile/controlling caregiving might differentially affect neurophysiological development relative to emotionally neglectful/unresponsive caregiving. Across levels of ecological influence, the presence of protective or vulnerability factors related to socioeconomic status, parenting quality, social support, and culture may moderate the relation between adversity and adaptation (Yates & Masten, 2004). Finally, the child's genetic constitution, developmental history, and the quality of her/his current adaptation (e.g., comorbid psychopathology) may influence the relation between CEA exposure and response (Cicchetti & Rogosch, 2001b; Kaufman et al., 1997; Sapolsky, 1994). As our understanding of the impact of adversity on neurobiological development and adaptation advances, we must achieve similar gains in our recognition of factors that moderate observed relations among adversity, neurodevelopment, and socioemotional adaptation.

Fourth, in keeping with the call for greater attention to moderating variables in future research, a developmental psychopathology framework encourages attention not only to processes that engender risk, but also to those that confer strength in the face of vulnerability. Just as psychobiological processes may contribute to maladaptation, so, too, may they underlie the better-than-expected processes and outcomes that typify resilience (Curtis & Cicchetti, 2003; Davidson, 2000). Research aimed at identifying both positive and pathological pathways following CEA will further our understanding of specific processes underlying observed patterns. Indeed, the salience of parenting quality for the developing stress response system was revealed only by the study of the better-than-expected outcomes that followed from early handling paradigms. As observed by Curtis and Cicchetti (2003), such research may profitably explore whether positive adaptation in the face of adversity derives from greater resistance to adversity, greater resources for recovery, and/or greater capacity for compensation.

As a macroparadigm, developmental psychopathology is uniquely equipped to bridge artificial dualisms between different lenses of empirical inquiry, between behavioral and biological science, and between basic and applied research. Building on this framework, future research must adopt interdisciplinary, integrative paradigms that can be readily translated to real-world practice with children and families. In addition to the adoption of a developmental psychopathology framework, there must be an appreciation for interdisciplinary collaborations at the level of funding agencies and professional evaluative networks. In short, an individualistic science of psychology cannot uncover the dynamic multisystem transactions that underlie development and adaptation. Future research must transcend single-level designs (e.g., including both biological and socioemotional assessments) and incorporate multiple methods and measures within levels (e.g., including several indicators of physiological functioning, such as cortisol, catecholamines, neuroelectrical activity and neuroimaging). Undoubtedly, this work rests at the precipice of psychology's growing edge (see Nelson et al., 2002 for a discussion of issues and examples of this kind of work). However, understanding the relations between adversity and neural development, and identifying factors that moderate these relations, holds tremendous promise for intervention efforts aimed at reducing the deleterious impact of early adversity.

Directions for Future Practice

Relative to interventions targeting physically and sexually abused children, and to a lesser degree neglected children, there has been little attention directed toward helping emotionally abused children. Psychotherapeutic and/or pharmacological interventions may prevent or reverse the deleterious effects of early stress exposure at both behavioral and physiological levels (Curtis & Nelson, 2003; Kandel, 1998; Nelson, 2000). Just as plasticity renders the organism vulnerable to deviations in adaptive processes, so, too, does it confer a capacity for resistance, self-righting, and recovery. Adopting a developmental psychopathology perspective in research on both positive and pathological pathways following exposure to CEA has important implications for the design and implementation of effective intervention efforts, especially in terms of identifying particular populations, and systems within them, to target.

One implication of this approach is that periods of rapid development harbinger greater vulnerability to both positive and negative influences. As such, childhood, with its attendant elevation in neural growth and modification, may be an especially vulnerable period, either to the degenerative effects of maltreatment or to the restorative effects of intervention. That being said, the potential for psychobiological plasticity extends well into adulthood such that the human brain continues to respond to both positive (e.g., training) and negative (e.g., injury) experiences over the life course (Nelson & Bloom, 1997). Although it is important for intervention efforts to target core developmental systems in early childhood, the inclusion of follow-up supports will be important for the maintenance of positive gains over time.

Preclinical and clinical studies suggest that the caregiving system may be especially influential in the prevention, amelioration, or reversal of negative consequences related to CEA. Animal studies demonstrate that environmental factors (e.g., social enrichment, improved caregiving) can modulate neurogenerative and stress response processes (Francis, Diorio et al., 1999; Liu et al., 1997). In humans, attachment security, which is a proxy for sensitive and responsive caregiving, buffers human stress response systems (Gunnar, 1998; Nachmias et al., 1996). The attachment system is a profitable target for intervention because it carries the possibility for both protective and restorative processes at multiple levels of action (see Egeland, Weinfield, Bosquet, & Cheng, 2000 for review). In a recent intervention study, Fisher and colleagues (2000) demonstrated the efficacy of early intervention (EI) efforts focused on the quality of the child-caregiver relationship for both behavioral and physiological aspects of development. In this study, a group of maltreated preschoolers (sexual abuse, physical abuse, exposure to partner violence and other trauma) were placed in an EI foster care program that consisted of foster parent education, child and family therapy, and parent support groups intended to encourage consistent (nonabusive) discipline, positive reinforcement, and close monitoring of the child. After 12 weeks of treatment, behavioral effects were found for both foster parents and children. The EI group exhibited improved parenting practices relative to regular foster care parents. In addition, the children in the EI group evidenced notable declines in symptom endorsement on an inventory of child behavior problems, while children in the regular foster care group evidenced progressive increases in behavioral maladaptation. Salivary cortisol measures indicated that the EI children exhibited a significant shift toward normative circadian cortisol release over the course of treatment, whereas children in regular foster care exhibited increasingly atypical patterns. Although preliminary in nature, these findings suggest that early intervention and prevention efforts may prove integral to socioemotional *and* neurophysiological adaptation and recovery (see Dozier, Lindheim, & Ackerman, 2005 for review).

As evident in the EI program described above, successful intervention with high-risk families requires a multi-faceted approach to service provision that aims to support and restore core adaptational systems, such as the attachment relationship (see Erickson, 1998 for discussion). To this end, efforts to prevent CEA and support positive parenting might include services to reduce caregiver strain (e.g., economic, educational, occupational resources), improve caregiver understanding of child development (e.g., parent education, parent sensitivity training), and foster social networks that can maintain positive change beyond the parameters of a particular intervention (e.g., home visitation, support groups). Just as pathology derives from multiple levels of influence, so, too, must intervention efforts transcend these levels to foster positive developmental outcomes.

Developmentally appropriate, systems-oriented, multi-pronged prevention and intervention efforts will emerge out of interdisciplinary collaborations between scholars and practitioners, between animal and human researchers, and between scientists and the communities they serve. Historically, interdisciplinary and translational endeavors of this kind have been stymied by overemphasis on specialization and individual achievement in training and funding organizations. However, there is a growing recognition that the inclusion of diverse sources of information, such as evaluation research or biological measures of development and adaptation, not only informs interventions, but also affirms, expands, and challenges extant theories about adversity and adaptation (Cicchetti & Hinshaw, 2002; Yates & Masten, 2004).

CONCLUDING COMMENTS

CEA disrupts development across multiple domains, including social, emotional, self, cognitive, and biological processes. Although research has heretofore focused almost exclusively on psychological mechanisms in understanding pathways from CEA to various outcomes, evidence indicates that CEA has the capacity to initiate persistent alterations in neurophysiological stress response systems that lead to increased vulnerability for stress, anxiety, depression, and other problems of adaptation. In order to better understand these processes and identify meaningful ways to intervene, research and practice must draw on multiple levels of analysis across theoretical, empirical, and applied domains. The integrative paradigm of developmental psychopathology provides a conceptual framework that can bridge prior factions between science and practice and between developmental psychology and neurobiology.

Understanding the psychobiological correlates and consequences of child maltreatment broadly, and CEA in particular, has significant importance for future research and programming aimed at mitigating or reversing its negative impact on development, as well as for potentially preventing its transmission to subsequent generations. As reviewed here, a preponderance of evidence indicates that "adequate nurturance and the absence of intense early stress permits our brains to develop in a manner that is less aggressive and more emotionally stable, social, empathic and hemispherically integrated" (Teicher, 2002, p. 75). This article encourages and informs the development and implementation of multi-faceted, developmentally informed interventions that encompass multiple levels of change and adaptation to foster basic adaptational systems that buffer and scaffold physiological and psychological development.

REFERENCES

American Professional Society on the Abuse of Children. (1995). *Psychosocial evaluation of suspected psychological maltreatment in children and adolescents: Practice guidelines*. Chicago, IL: American Professional Society on the Abuse of Children.

Behl, L. E., Conyngham, H. A., & May, P. F. (2003). Trends in child maltreatment literature. *Child Abuse and Neglect, 27*, 215-229.

Bremner, J. D. (1999). Does stress damage the brain? *Biological Psychiatry, 45*, 797-805.

Bremner, J. D., Krystal, J. H., Sowthwick, S. M., & Charney, D. S. (1996). Noradrenergic mechanism in stress and anxiety: II. Clinical studies. *Synapse, 23*, 39-51.

Bremner, J. D., & Vermetten, E. (2001). Stress and development: Behavioral and biological consequences. *Development and Psychopathology, 13*, 473-489.

Briere, J., & Runtz, M. (1988). Multivariate correlates of childhood psychological and physical maltreatment among university women. *Child Abuse and Neglect, 12*, 331-341.

Bugental, D. B., Martorell, G. A., & Barazza, V. (2003). The hormonal costs of subtle forms of infant maltreatment. *Hormones and Behavior, 43*, 237-244.

Bugental, D. B., Olster, D. H., & Martorell, G. A. (2003). A developmental neuroscience perspective on the dynamics of parenting. In L. Kuczynski (Ed.), *Handbook of dynamics in parent-child relations* (pp. 25-48). Thousand Oaks, CA: Sage Publications.

Cacioppo, J. T., & Berntson, G. G. (1992). Social psychological contributions to the decade of the brain: Doctrine of multilevel analysis. *American Psychologist, 47*(8), 1019-1028.

Caldji, C., Diorio, J., & Meaney, M. J. (2000). Variations in maternal care in infancy regulate the development of stress reactivity. *Biological Psychiatry, 48*, 1164-1174.

Caldji, C., Tannenbaum, B., Sharma, S., Francis, D., Plotsky, P. M., & Meaney, M. J. (1998). Maternal care during infancy regulates the development of neural systems mediating the expression of fearfulness in the rat. *Proceedings of the National Academy of Sciences, 95*, 5335-5340.

Chrousos, G. P. (1998). Stressors, stress, and neuroendocrine integration of the adaptive response: The 1997 Hans Selye Memorial Lecture. *Annals of the New York Academy of Sciences, 851*, 311-335.

Cicchetti, D. (1993). Developmental psychopathology: Reactions, reflections, projection. *Developmental Review, 13*, 471-502.

Cicchetti, D. (2003). Neuroendocrine functioning in maltreated children. In D. Cicchetti & E. F. Walker (Eds.), *Neurodevelopmental mechanisms in psychopathology* (pp. 345-365). New York: Cambridge University Press.

Cicchetti, D., & Blender, J. A. (2004). A multiple-levels-of-analysis approach to the study of developmental processes in maltreated children. *Proceedings of the National Academy of Sciences, 101*(50), 17325-17326.

Cicchetti, D., & Hinshaw, S. P. (Eds.). (2002). *Development and Psychopathology, special issue: Prevention and intervention science: Contributions to developmental theory* (Vol. 14). New York: Cambridge University Press.

Cicchetti, D., & Nurcombe, B. (Eds.). (1991). *Development and Psychopathology, special issue: Defining psychological maltreatment: Reflections and future directions* (Vol. 3). New York: Cambridge University Press.

Cicchetti, D., & Rogosch, F. A. (2001a). Diverse patterns of neuroendocrine activity in maltreated children. *Development and Psychopathology, 13*, 677-694.

Cicchetti, D., & Rogosch, F. A. (2001b). The impact of child maltreatment and psychopathology upon neuroendocrine functioning. *Development and Psychopathology, 13*, 783-804.

Cicchetti, D., & Toth, S. L. (1997). Transactional ecological systems in developmental psychopathology. In S. S. Luthar, J. A. Burack, D. Cicchetti & J. R. Weisz (Eds.), *Developmental psychopathology: Perspectives on adjustment, risk, and disorder* (pp. 317-349). New York: Cambridge University Press.

Cicchetti, D., & Toth, S. L. (2000). Developmental processes in maltreated children. In D. J. Hansen (Ed.), *Nebraska symposium on motivation: Child maltreatment* (Vol. 46, pp. 85-160). Lincoln, NE: University of Nebraska Press.

Cicchetti, D., & Walker, M. (Eds.). (2003). *Neurodevelopmental mechanisms in psychopathology*. New York: Cambridge University Press.

Claussen, A., & Crittenden, P. M. (1991). Physical and psychological maltreatment: Relations among types of maltreatment. *Child Abuse and Neglect, 15*, 5-18.

Coplan, J. D., Paunica, A. D., & Rosenblum, L. A. (2004). Neuropsychobiology of the variable foraging demand paradigm in nonhuman primates. In J. M. Gorman (Ed.), *Fear and anxiety: The benefits of translational research* (pp. 47-64). Washington, DC: American Psychiatric Publishing, Inc.

Curtis, J. W., & Cicchetti, D. (2003). Moving research on resilience into the 21st century: Theoretical and methodological considerations in examining the biological contributors to resilience. *Development and Psychopathology, 15*, 773-810.

Curtis, J. W., & Nelson, C. A. (2003). Toward building a better brain: Neurobehavioral outcomes, mechanisms, and processes of environmental enrichment. In S. Luthar (Ed.), *Resilience and vulnerability: Adaptation in the context of childhood adversities* (pp. 463-488). New York: Cambridge University Press.

Davidson, R. J. (2000). Affective style, psychopathology, and resilience: Brain mechanisms and plasticity. *American Psychologist, 55*, 1196-1214.

De Bellis, M. D., Baum, A. S., Birmaher, B., Keshavan, M. S., Eccard, C. H., Boring, A. M. et al. (1999). Developmental traumatology Part I: Biological stress systems. *Biological Psychiatry, 45*(10), 1259-1270.

De Bellis, M. D., Keshavan, M. S., Clark, D. B., Casey, B. J., Giedd, J. N., Boring, A. M., et al. (1999). Developmental traumatology Part II: Brain development. *Biological Psychiatry, 45*(10), 1271-1284.

De Bellis, M. D., & Putnam, F. W. (1994). The psychobiology of childhood maltreatment. *Child and Adolescent Psychiatric Clinics of North America, 3*, 663-677.

Dettling, A. C., Parker, S., Lane, S. K., Sebanc, A. M., & Gunnar, M. R. (2000). Quality of care and temperament determine whether cortisol levels rise over the day for children in full-day childcare. *Psychoneuroendocrinology, 25*, 819-836.

Dozier, M., Lindheim, O., & Ackerman, J. P. (2005). Attachment and biobehavioral catch-up: An intervention targeting empirically identified needs in foster infants. In L. J. Berlin, Y. Ziv, L. Amaya-Jackson & M. T. Greenberg (Eds.), *Enhancing early attachments: Theory, research, intervention, and policy* (pp. 178-194). New York: Guilford.

Egeland, B., Weinfield, N. S., Bosquet, M., & Cheng, V. K. (2000). Remembering, repeating, and working through: Lessons from attachment-based interventions. In J. D. Osofsky & H. E. Fitzgerald (Eds.), *Infant mental health in groups at high risk. WAIMH handbook of infant mental health* (Vol. 4, pp. 35-89). New York: John Wiley & Sons, Inc.

Erickson, M. F. (1998). Strong beginnings: Promoting resiliency through secure parent-infant relationships. In K. Bogenschneider & J. Olson (Eds.), *Building resiliency and reducing risk: What youth need from families and communities to succeed* (Vol. 10, pp. 50-59). Madison, WI: University of Wisconsin Center for Excellence in Family Studies.

Erickson, M. F., Egeland, B., & Pianta, R. (1989). The effects of maltreatment on the development of young children. In D. Cicchetti & V. Carlson (Eds.), *Child maltreatment: Theory and research on the causes and consequences of child abuse and neglect* (pp. 647-684). New York: Cambridge University Press.

Fisher, P. A., Gunnar, M. R., Chamberlain, P., & Reid, J. B. (2000). Preventive intervention for maltreated preschool children: Impact on children's behavior, neuroendocrine activity, and foster parent functioning. *Journal of the American Academy of Child and Adolescent Psychiatry, 39*(11), 1356-1364.

Francis, D. D., Caldji, C., Champagne, F., Plotsky, P. M., & Meaney, M. J. (1999). The role of corticotropin-releasing factor norepinephrine systems in mediating the effects of early experience on the development of behavioral and endocrine responses to stress. *Biological Psychiatry, 46*, 1153-1166.

Francis, D. D., Diorio, J., Liu, D., & Meaney, M. J. (1999). Nongenomic transmission across generations of maternal behavior and stress responses in the rat. *Science, 286*(5442), 1155-1158.

Francis, D. D., & Meaney, M. J. (1999). Maternal care and development of stress responses. *Current Opinion in Neurobiology, 9*, 128-134.

Garrison, E. G. (1987). Psychological maltreatment of children: An emerging focus for inquiry and concern. *American Psychologist, 42*(2), 157-159.

Geffner, R., & Rossman, B. B. R. (1998). Emotional abuse: An emerging field of research and intervention. *Journal of Emotional Abuse, 1*, 1-5.

Glaser, D. (2000). Child abuse and neglect and the brain: A review. *Journal of Child Psychology and Psychiatry, 41*, 97-116.

Gottlieb, G., & Halpern, C. T. (2002). A relational view of causality in normal and abnormal development. *Development and Psychopathology, 14*, 421-435.

Granger, D. A., Weisz, J. R., McCracken, J. T., Ikeda, S. C., & Douglas, P. (1996). Reciprocal influences among adrenocortical activation, psychosocial processes, and the behavioral adjustment of clinic-referred children. *Child Development, 67*, 3250-3262.

Gross, A. B., & Keller, H. R. (1992). Long-term consequences of childhood physical and psychological maltreatment. *Aggressive Behavior, 18*, 171-185.

Gunnar, M. R. (1998). Quality of early care and buffering of neuroendocrine stress reactions: Potential effects on the developing human brain. *Preventive Medicine, 27*, 208-211.

Gunnar, M. R., Brodersen, L., Nachmias, M., Buss, K., & Rigatuso, J. (1996). Stress reactivity and attachment security. *Developmental Psychobiology, 29*(3), 191-204.

Gunnar, M. R., Broderson, L., Krueger, K., & Rigatuso, J. (1996). Dampening of adrenocortical responses during infancy: Normative changes and individual differences. *Child Development, 67*, 877-889.

Gunnar, M. R., & Cheatham, C. L. (2003). Brain and behavior interface: Stress and the developing brain. *Infant Mental Health Journal, 24*(3), 195-211.

Gunnar, M. R., Larson, M., Hertsgaard, L., Harris, M., & Brodersen, L. (1992). The stressfulness of separation among 9-month-old infants: Effects on social context variables and infant temperament. *Child Development, 63*, 290-303.

Gunnar, M. R., Tout, K., deHaan, M., Pierce, S., & Stansbury, K. (1997). Temperament, social competence, and adrenocortical activity in preschoolers. *Developmental Psychobiology, 31*, 65-85.

Hart, J., Gunnar, M. R., & Cicchetti, D. (1995). Salivary cortisol levels in maltreated children: Evidence of relations between neuroendocrine activity and social competence. *Development and Psychopathology, 7*, 11-26.

Hart, S. N., Binggeli, N. J., & Brassard, M. R. (1998). Evidence for the effects of psychological maltreatment. *Journal of Emotional Abuse, 1*, 27-58.

Hart, S. N., Brassard, M. R., Binggeli, N. J., & Davidson, H. A. (2001). Psychological maltreatment. In J. E. B. Myers, L. Berliner, J. Briere, C. T. Hendrix, C. Jenny & T. A. Reid (Eds.), *The APSAC Handbook on Child Maltreatment* (2nd ed., pp. 79-103). Thousand Oaks, CA: Sage Publications.

Heim, C., Ehlert, U., & Hellhammer, D. (2000). The potential role of hypocortisolism in the pathophysiology of stress-related bodily disorders. *Psychoneuroendocrinology, 25*, 1-35.

Heim, C., & Nemeroff, C. B. (2001). The role of childhood trauma in the neurobiology of mood and anxiety disorders: Preclinical and clinical studies. *Biological Psychiatry, 49*, 1023-1039.

Heim, C., Owen, M. J., Plotsky, P. M., & Nemeroff, C. B. (1997). The role of early life events in the etiology of depression and posttraumatic stress disorder: Focus on corticotropin releasing factor. *Annals of the New York Academy of Sciences, 821*, 194-207.

Herrenkohl, R. C., Herrenkohl, E. C., Egolf, B., & Wu, P. (1991). The developmental consequences of child abuse: The Lehigh longitudinal study. In R. H. Starr & D. Wolfe (Eds.), *The effects of child abuse and neglect: Issues and research* (pp. 57-80). New York: Guilford Publications.

Hertsgaard, L., Gunnar, M. R., Erickson, M. F., & Nachmias, M. (1995). Adrenocortical responses to the Strange Situation in infants with disorganized/disoriented attachment relationships. *Child Development, 66*, 1100-1106.

Iwaniec, D. (1995). *The emotionally abused and neglected child: Identification, assessment and intervention*. New York: John Wiley & Sons.

Johnson, J. G., Cohen, P., Smailes, E. M., Skodol, A. E., Brown, J., & Oldham, J. M. (2001). Childhood verbal abuse and risk for personality disorders during adolescence and early adulthood. *Comprehensive Psychiatry, 42*, 16-23.

Jones, N. A., Field, T., Fox, N. A., Davalos, M., Malphurs, J., Carraway, K., et al. (1997). Infants of intrusive and withdrawn mothers. *Infant Behavior & Development, 20*(2), 175-186.

Kandel, E. R. (1998). A new intellectual framework for psychiatry. *American Journal of Psychiatry, 155*, 469-475.

Kaufman, J., Birmaher, B., Perel, J., Dahl, R. E., Moreci, P., Nelson, B., et al. (1997). The corticotropin-releasing hormone challenge in depressed abused, depressed nonabused, and normal control children. *Biological Psychiatry, 42*, 669-679.

Kaufman, J., Plotsky, P. M., Nemeroff, C. B., & Charney, D. (2000). Effects of early adverse experiences on brain structure and function: Clinical implications. *Biological Psychiatry, 48*, 778-790.

Kempe, C. H., Silverman, F. N., Steele, B. F., Droegemueller, W., & Silver, H. K. (1962). The battered-child syndrome. *Journal of the American Medical Association, 251*, 3288-3300.

Kolb, L. (1989). Brain development, plasticity, and behavior. *American Psychologist, 44*, 1203-1212.

Koob, G. F. (1999). Corticotropin-releasing factor, norepinephrine, and stress. *Biological Psychiatry, 46*, 1167-1180.

Ladd, C. O., Owens, M., & Nemeroff, C. B. (1996). Persistent changes in corticotropin-releasing factor neuronal systems induced by maternal deprivation. *Endocrinology, 137*, 1212-1218.

Levine, S. (2001). Primary social relationships influence the development of the hypothalamic-pituitary-adrenal axis in the rat. *Physiological Behavior, 13*, 255-260.

Liu, D., Diorio, J., Tannenbaum, B., Caldji, C., Rancis, D., Freedman, A., et al. (1997). Maternal care, hippocampal glucocorticoid receptors, and hypothalamic-pituitary-adrenal responses to stress. *Science, 277*, 1659-1662.

Lopez, J. F., Akil, H., & Watson, S. J. (1999). Neural circuits mediating stress. *Biological Psychiatry, 46*, 1461-1471.

Manly, J. T., Kim, J. E., Rogosch, F. A., & Cicchetti, D. (2001). Dimensions of child maltreatment and children's adjustment: Contributions of developmental timing and subtype. *Development and Psychopathology, 13*, 759-782.

Margolin, G., & Gordis, E. B. (2000). The effects of family and community violence on children. *Annual Review of Psychology, 51*, 445-479.

Masten, A. S. (2006). Developmental psychopathology: Pathways to the future. *International Journal of Behavioral Development, 31*(1), 38-45.

McEwen, B. S. (2000). Allostasis and allostatic load: Implications for neuropsychopharmacology. *Neuropsychopharmacology, 22*(2), 108-124.

Mullen, P. E., Martin, J. L., Anderson, J. C., Romans, S. E., & Herbison, G. P. (1996). The long-term impact of the physical, emotional, and sexual abuse of children: A community study. *Child Abuse and Neglect, 20*, 7-21.

Nachmias, M., Gunnar, M. R., Mangelsdorf, S., Parritz, R. H., & Buss, K. (1996). Behavioral inhibition and stress reactivity: The moderating role of attachment security. *Child Development, 67*, 508-522.

Navarre, E. L. (1987). Psychological maltreatment: The core component of child abuse. In M. R. Brassard, R. Germain & S. N. Hart (Eds.), *Psychological maltreatment of children and youth* (pp. 45-56). New York: Pergamon Press.

Nelson, C. A. (2000). The neurobiological bases of early intervention. In J. P. Shonkoff & S. J. Meisels (Eds.), *Handbook of early childhood intervention* (2nd ed., pp. 204-227). New York: Cambridge University Press.

Nelson, C. A., & Bloom, F. E. (1997). Child development and neuroscience. *Child Development, 68*, 970-987.

Nelson, C. A., Bloom, F. E., Cameron, J. L., Amaral, D., Dahl, R. E., & Pine, D. S. (2002). An integrative, multidisciplinary approach to the study of brain-behavior relations in the context of typical and atypical development. *Development and Psychopathology, 14*, 599-520.

Nelson, C. A., & Carver, L. J. (1998). The effects of stress and trauma on brain and memory: A view from developmental cognitive neuroscience. *Development and Psychopathology, 10*, 793-810.

Nemeroff, C. B. (2004). Neurobiological consequences of childhood trauma. *Journal of Clinical Psychiatry, 65*(suppl. 1), 18-28.

Owens, M., & Nemeroff, C. B. (1991). Physiology and pharmacology of corticotropin-releasing factor. *Pharmacological Review, 43*, 425-473.

Perry, B. D., & Pollard, R. A. (1998). Homeostasis, stress, trauma, and adaptation: A neurodevelopmental view of childhood trauma. *Child and Adolescent Psychiatric Clinics of North America, 7*, 33-51.

Plotsky, P. M., & Meaney, M. J. (1993). Early, postnatal experience alters hypothalamic corticotropin-relasing factor (CRF) mRNA, median eminence CRF content and stress-induced release in rats. *Brain Research and Molecular Brain Research, 18*, 195-200.

Roozendal, B., Koolhaas, J. M., & Bohus, K. (1997). The role of the central amygdala in stress and adaptation. *Acta Physiologica Scandinavia Supplement, 640*, 51-54.

Sanchez, M. M., Ladd, C. O., & Plotsky, P. M. (2001). Early adverse experience as a developmental risk factor for later psychopathology: Evidence from rodent and primate models. *Development and Psychopathology, 13*, 419-450.

Sapolsky, R. M. (1994). Individual differences and the stress response. *Seminars in the Neurosciences, 6*, 261-269.

Sapolsky, R. M. (1996). Stress, glucocorticoids, and damage to the NS: The current state of confusion. *Stress, 1*, 1-19.

Solomon, R., & Serres, F. (1999). Effects of parental verbal aggression on children's self-esteem and school marks. *Child Abuse and Neglect, 23*(4), 339-351.

Spangler, G., & Grossman, K. E. (1993). Biobehavioral organization in securely and insecurely attached infants. *Child Development, 64*, 1439-1450.

Spertus, I. L., Yehuda, R., Wong, C. M., Halligan, S., & Seremetis, S. V. (2003). Childhood emotional abuse and neglect as predictors of psychological and physical symptoms in women presenting to a primary care practice. *Child Abuse and Neglect, 27*, 1247-1258.

Sroufe, L. A., & Rutter, M. (1984). The domain of developmental psychopathology. *Child Development, 55*, 17-29.

Teicher, M. H. (2002). Scars that won't heal: The neurobiology of child abuse. *Scientific American, 286*(3), 68-76.

Valentino, R. J., Curtis, A. L., Page, M. E., Pavcovich, L. A., & Florin-Lechner, S. M. (1998). Activation of the locus ceruleus brain noradrenergic system during stress: Circuitry, consequences, and regulation. *Advances in Pharmacology, 42*, 781-784.

Vasquez, D. M. (1998). Stress and the developing limbic-hypothalamic-pituitary-adrenal axis. *Psychoneuroendocrinology, 23*, 663-700.

Vissing, Y. M., Straus, M. A., Gelles, R. J., & Harrop, J. W. (1991). Verbal aggression by parents and psychosocial problems of children. *Child Abuse and Neglect, 15*, 223-238.

Yates, T. M., & Masten, A. S. (2004). Fostering the future: Resilience theory and the practice of positive psychology. In P. A. Linley & S. Joseph (Eds.), *Positive Psychology in Practice* (pp. 521-539). Hoboken, NJ: John Wiley and Sons, Inc.

Yehuda, R., Halligan, S. L., & Grossman, R. (2001). Childhood trauma and risk for PTSD: Relationship to intergenerational effects of trauma, parental PTSD, and cortisol excretion. *Development and Psychopathology, 13*, 733-753.

Yehuda, R., Southwick, S. M., Mason, J. W., & Giller, E. L. (1990). Interactions of the hypothalamic-pituitary-adrenal axis and the catecholaminergic system of the stress disorder. In E. L. Giller (Ed.), *Biological assessment and treatment of PTSD*. Washington, DC: American Psychiatric Press.

doi:10.1300/J135v07n02_02

Cardiovascular Correlates of Interpersonal Mistreatment in Healthy Adults

Tamara L. Newton
Rebecca A. Weigel

SUMMARY. The present study examined connections between self-reported experiences of interpersonal mistreatment and cardiovascular responses during laboratory dyadic interactions. One hundred and eight unacquainted participants were paired to form 54 opposite-gender, same-ethnicity (22 African American and 32 European American) dyads. Blood pressure and heart rate responses were monitored while dyads participated in three 4-minute problem-solving focused interactions. Multilevel modeling revealed significant, positive associations between frequency of interpersonal mistreatment and systolic and diastolic resting blood pressure levels among African American men and European American women. Among all women, significant and positive associations were observed between mistreatment and diastolic blood pressure reactivity assessed during the problem-solving focused interactions. Results

Address correspondence to: Tamara L. Newton, Department of Psychological and Brain Sciences, University of Louisville, Belknap Campus, 317 Life Sciences Building, Louisville, KY 40292 (E-mail: tlnewton@louisville.edu).

This work was supported by NHLBI R29 HL58528, awarded to the first author.

[Haworth co-indexing entry note]: "Cardiovascular Correlates of Interpersonal Mistreatment in Healthy Adults." Newton, Tamara L., and Rebecca A. Weigel. Co-published simultaneously in *Journal of Emotional Abuse* (The Haworth Maltreatment & Trauma Press, an imprint of The Haworth Press. Inc.) Vol. 7, No. 2, 2007, pp. 35-58; and: *Childhood Emotional Abuse: Mediating and Moderating Processes Affecting Long-Term Impact* (ed: Margaret O'Dougherty Wright) The Haworth Maltreatment & Trauma Press, an imprint of The Haworth Press, Inc.. 2007, pp. 35-58. Single or multiple copies of this article are available for a fee from The Haworth Document Delivery Service [1-800-HAWORTH, 9:00 a.m. - 5:00 p.m. (EST). E-mail address: docdelivery@haworthpress.com].

Available online at http://jea.haworthpress.com

doi:10.1300/J135v07n02_03

highlight interpersonal mistreatment as a potential contributor to cardiovascular functioning for both men and women. doi:10.1300/J135v07n02_03

KEYWORDS. Interpersonal mistreatment, blood pressure, cardiovascular reactivity, gender, ethnicity

INTRODUCTION

The cardiovascular system is a dynamic system, enabling individuals to adaptively respond to alterations in environmental circumstances (Sterling & Eyer, 1988). Some cardiovascular changes occur in response to metabolic requirements triggered by shifts in posture, activity, and states of arousal, such as sleep versus wakefulness (Pickering & Kario, 2001; Sterling & Eyer, 1988). Other cardiovascular changes, and those that are the focus of the present study, are a function of psychological circumstances, such as emotional qualities of the social environment (Seeman & McEwen, 1996).

Of interest in the present study are associations between cardiovascular functioning and negative emotional aspects of the social environment. Although studies in this area have used diverse paradigms and have assessed cardiovascular correlates of a variety of interpersonal events, all such events can be characterized as negatively valenced socio-emotional experiences. Collectively, these experiences have been referred to as "relational adversity" (Seeman, Singer, Ryff, Love, & Levy-Storms, 2002, p. 396), although they lie along a spectrum of severity. For example, some studies in this area have examined associations between cardiovascular functioning and severe negative interpersonal experiences, such as potentially traumatic interpersonal abuse and victimization (Murali & Chen, 2005; Newton, Parker, & Ho, 2005). Other studies have examined negative interpersonal experiences that are less severe (e.g., conflict between relatively happily married couples; Newton & Sanford, 2003) but have potentially important cardiovascular consequences nonetheless. In the present study, we examined cardiovascular correlates of self-reported experiences of interpersonal mistreatment (Guyll, Matthews, & Bromberger, 2001; Williams, Yu, & Jackson, 1997). Such mistreatment encompasses exposure to hostile social interactions and to actions that either implicitly or explicitly communicate disrespect and affront one's social worth or rank.

It is well established that direct exposure to negative social interactions, even those that are apparently benign and commonplace enough to be ethically studied in the laboratory, has consequences for blood pressure and heart rate. For example, greater blood pressure reactivity is apparent in adults facing an acute stressor in an emotionally cold and potentially punitive social context, compared to a low social threat context (Kamarck, Annunziato, & Amateau, 1995), as well as in an indifferent social environment, compared to facing the stressor alone (Lepore, Mata, & Evans, 1993). In addition, significant elevations in blood pressure accompany expression of, and exposure to, hostility and dominance in interactions between adult strangers (Newton & Bane, 2001) and between close partners (Brown, Smith, & Benjamin, 1998; Ewart, Taylor, Kraemer, & Agras, 1991; Newton & Sanford, 2003), with some evidence that these connections are more consistent for women than men (Ewart et al., 1991).

Other studies reveal physiological consequences of negative social experiences beyond those due to direct exposure. For example, simply recalling and recounting adverse social relationships, compared to supportive, indifferent, and ambivalent relationships, generates significant blood pressure reactivity. This effect was apparent among women, but not men (Bloor, Uchino, Hicks, & Smith, 2004). In addition, one study offers preliminary evidence that exposure to interpersonal mistreatment may carry over to influence cardiovascular responses to subsequent situations. Specifically, reports of frequent interpersonal mistreatment characterized by subtle disrespect were associated with elevated resting heart rate among European American women and with elevated diastolic blood pressure reactivity to acute laboratory stressors among African American women (Guyll et al., 2001). In contrast, reports of frequent mistreatment characterized by blatant threats and accusations were associated with lower resting heart rate among African American women (Guyll et al., 2001). Although in this preliminary investigation reasons for the mixed pattern of results were unclear, it is relevant to note that both hyper- and hypo-responsivity of the cardiovascular system have been observed in studies of other life stressors (Gump & Matthews, 1999; Murali & Chen, 2005).

During actual negative social interactions, cardiovascular activation may be considered an expected, or even adaptive, response that subserves the action tendencies and behavioral strategies associated with emotional states provoked by clear and present social threats (Lovallo, 2005). Over the long term, however, physiological costs may accrue. In a sample of older adults between the ages of 70 and 79, reports of frequent demands and criticisms from one's spouse were associated with elevations in a cumulative biological indicator of all-cause mortality risk encompassing levels of basal blood pressure, urinary endocrine hormones, lipoproteins, and other biobehavioral measures (Seeman et al., 2002). A non-significant trend for stronger associations among women than men was noted. Additionally, in a sample of otherwise healthy African American women, interpersonal mistreatment, characterized by a combination of both subtle disrespect and blatant threats and accusations, was significantly and positively associated with carotid artery intima-media thickness, an indicator of subclinical carotid artery disease. This association held after controlling for the effects for major life events and economic hardship (Troxel, Matthews, Bromberger, & Sutton-Tyrrell, 2003). Similarly, a recent longitudinal study observed that chronic mistreatment experienced over the course of five years is associated with increased likelihood of coronary artery calcification among mid-life African American women (Lewis et al., 2006). Taken together, these studies provide preliminary evidence for longer term health consequences of negatively valenced socioemotional experiences. In addition, by providing a mechanism for recurrent and sustained physiological activation even in the absence of direct exposure to negative social experiences, the physiological carry over described above may also be construed as a longer term cost of such experiences.

The purpose of the present study was to further examine the cardiovascular psychophysiology of adverse social experiences, and specifically, interpersonal mistreatment. Building on the research of Guyll et al. (2001), we utilized a laboratory paradigm to examine cardiovascular correlates of interpersonal mistreatment and extended existing research by assessing heart rate and blood pressure during brief, problem-solving focused dyadic interactions. As potentially stressful social situations, these interactions provided a relevant context for assessing the cardiovascular functioning of individuals who have experienced interpersonal mistreatment. As outcomes, we examined cardiovascular reactivity and cardiovascular resting levels, two response patterns that have been hypothesized to partially mediate connections between a variety of stressors, including those of a social nature, and long term negative health outcomes (McEwen, 1998). Finally, whereas the one prior study of interpersonal mistreatment and cardiovascular functioning included women only, we included both men and women.

Although there is limited research on interpersonal mistreatment and cardiovascular functioning, we advanced the following hypotheses by extrapolating from the broader supporting literature reviewed above. First, we predicted that interpersonal mistreatment would be positively associated with resting cardiovascular levels. Second, we predicted that interpersonal mistreatment would be positively associated with cardiovascular reactivity to laboratory social interactions. Third, given the observed gender differences in this general research area, we predicted that associations with both levels and reactivity would be strongest for women.

Finally, we had two subsidiary aims. First, because Guyll et al. (2001) observed that associations between interpersonal mistreatment and cardiovascular responses varied by African American and European American ethnicity, we explored the potential contributions of ethnicity in the present study. Second, we considered the role of trait hostility in relationships between interpersonal mistreatment and cardiovascular reactivity. Hostile individuals are mistrustful of, and cynical about, the social world and may therefore have a greater propensity to perceive and react to instances of mistreatment. They also show elevated cardiovascular reactivity, particularly in social contexts (Suls & Wan, 1993). Therefore, we examined associations between interpersonal mistreatment and trait hostility and evaluated the contributions of mistreatment to cardiovascular responses above and beyond those of trait hostility.

METHOD

Participant Recruitment and Screening

Fifty-four women (22 African American, 32 European American) and 54 men (22 African American, 32 European American) were paired to participate in three 4-minute laboratory problem-solving focused interactions with one opposite-gender, same-ethnicity partner. The 108 participants were selected by screening 389 callers recruited by community advertisements as part of a larger investigation on gender, interpersonal processes, and health. For the purposes of limiting the sample to healthy African American and European American men and premenopausal women, a brief phone interview confirmed the following eligibility criteria: self-identified as either European-American, African-American, or biracial or multiethnic with African ancestry; between the ages of 18 and 35; no past or present cardiovascular-related medical conditions (e.g., hypertension, diabetes, renal disease); no current prescription medications for cardiovascular disorders or with significant cardiovascular side effects (except hormonal contraceptives); no history of a hospital stay for a psychiatric or emotional condition; and, for women, premenopausal status with at least one menstrual cycle within the last 12 months, and not currently pregnant or breastfeeding. In addition, for purposes of the broader investigation, only individuals who reported having one biological parent diagnosed with or treated for high blood pressure were eligible.

Laboratory Procedure

Participants were requested to refrain from caffeine, nicotine, and strenuous exercise for three hours prior to the session. They were scheduled for laboratory sessions in opposite-gender, same-ethnicity pairs, matched for age within five years. Each participant was greeted individually upon arrival and completed informed consent. Afterwards, participants were escorted to the lab, where they were introduced and it was confirmed that they were previously unacquainted. An occluding blood pressure cuff was placed over the brachial artery of each participant's non-dominant arm. In preparation for the discussions, each participant rated the strength of his or her opinions (0 = low, 7 = high) on 22 different potential discussion topics. Topics spanned a range of current events and social issues (e.g., pollution, gun control, affirmative action, health care). For discussion, the experimenter selected the three topics that were most highly rated by both participants (4 or above out of 7) and for which partners' ratings were most similar.

The laboratory session commenced with a 10-minute baseline, or initial rest. During this and all subsequent rests, a curtain was drawn between partners to prevent eye contact while they sat quietly. Following baseline, partners participated in three 4-minute videotaped interactions; the second and third discussions were each preceded by 10-minute interim rests. Multiple discussions were used because aggregating physiological assessments across measurement occasions enhances reliability and also enhances validity in the form of stronger relationships with individual difference measures (Epstein, 1984; Kamarck, 1992). Immediately prior to the start of each discussion, partners were presented with a topic and instructed to use the discussion period to arrive at a mutual decision regarding the three best ways to address the topic at hand. For purposes of the broader investigation of gender and stress reactivity, half of the dyads were assigned to a "maximal" (versus "typical") dominance condition by instructing both partners to be as dominant, influential, and assertive as possible. Assignment to dominance condition was balanced by ethnicity and gender. Because, for the present study, we advanced no hypotheses regarding this manipulation, condition was not included as a factor in statistical analyses and results therefore reflect responses aggregated across maximal and typical conditions. Following the third and final discussion, participants completed self-report measures in separate rooms and then received $35 for their participation.

Physiological Equipment and Measures

Systolic (SBP) and diastolic blood pressure (DBP) and heart rate (HR) were assessed using two Dinamap 8100 non-invasive blood pressure monitors (Critikon Corporation, Tampa, Florida). This monitor employs an oscillometric measurement method and possesses satisfactory reliability and accuracy when compared with intra-arterial measurements (Borow & Newberger, 1982). Cardiovascular readings were initiated at the beginning of minutes 3, 6, and 9 of the initial baseline, minutes 6 and 9 of the subsequent interim rests, and minutes 0 and 3 of all discussions. For each cardiovascular measure (i.e., SBP, DBP, HR), reactivity was assessed using change-scores calculated as the average for each discussion minus the average for the preceding rest, aggregated across the three discussions. Cardiovascular readings taken during the three rest periods were averaged to form an overall index of cardiovascular resting levels.

Psychosocial Measures

Interpersonal mistreatment. Participants rated 10 items to indicate how often (0 = never, 3 = often) they experienced interpersonal mistreatment characterized by subtle disrespect (e.g., others ignore you, act as if you are not smart) and blatant threats and accusations (e.g., you are threatened and harassed; Williams et al., 1997). Some studies have formed two subscales to distinguish between subtle disrespect (6 items) versus blatant threats and accusations (4 items) (e.g., Guyll et al., 2001), whereas others have generated a single mistreatment score (e.g., Lewis et al., 2006). In the present study, for tests of hypotheses, responses to the 10 items were summed to generate a single score, with higher scores reflecting more frequent experiences of mistreatment. This overall score has been positively associated with indicators of subclinical coronary artery disease among women (Lewis et al., 2006; Troxel et al., 2003). For descriptive purposes only, we generated separate subtle and blatant subscale scores to better understand the specific experiences of our participants. Cronbach's alpha for the 10-item scale was .87. For the subtle mistreatment subscale and the blatant mistreatment subscale, Cronbach's alphas were .85 and .76, respectively.

Cook and Medley Hostility Scale. Trait hostility was assessed by a 27-item short form of the Cook and Medley Hostility Scale, a better predictor of all-cause mortality than the original 50-item measure (Barefoot et al., 1989; Cook & Medley, 1954). These 27 true-false items, identified on rational and empirical bases, reflect the cynicism, hostile affect, and aggressive responding aspects of the larger scale (Barefoot et al., 1989). Sample items are "I have at times had to be rough with people who were rude or annoying" and "It is safer to trust nobody." The 1-year test-retest reliability of the 50-item scale among young adults is .85 (Barefoot, Dahlstrom, & Williams, 1983). Cronbach's alpha was .75 for the present sample.

State affect. Using 10-point scales (0 = low intensity, 9 = high intensity), participants rated 22 state affect descriptors after the initial baseline phase ("how you feel right now") and after each dyadic social interaction ("how you felt during the discussion"). For the present study, we focused on participants' reports of anger and fear, which we presumed would be most relevant to interpersonal mistreatment and cardiovascular functioning.

Sociodemographics and Health Characteristics

Height and weight were measured and used to calculate body mass index (kg/m^2). Standard demographic information (age, annual household income, and educational, marital, and occupational status) was collected by self-report. We also assessed smoking status (current smoker vs. non-smoker), caffeine consumption (at least weekly vs. less than weekly), and current use of hormonal contraceptives (i.e., oral, injected, or implanted).

Data Analytic Strategy

Multilevel modeling for dyadic data was used for analysis of cardiovascular resting levels, cardiovascular reactivity, and state affect baseline levels and change-scores (Campbell & Kashy, 2002). Models were run using SAS Proc Mixed, with restricted maximum likelihood estimation, and Satterthwaite approximation for degrees of freedom. This analytic approach circumvents the problem of non-independence of observations inherent in dyadic data by treating data from dyad members as two scores nested in a group where $n = 2$. On Step 1, trait hostility was entered as a covariate, and main effects of gender (coded 0 = women, 1 = men), ethnicity (coded 0 = European American, 1 = African American), and interpersonal mistreatment were tested. The three two-way interactions involving gender, ethnicity, and interpersonal mistreatment were tested in Step 2, and the three-way interaction of gender, ethnicity, and interpersonal mistreatment was tested in Step 3. Interpersonal mistreatment was centered around the grand mean, and product terms used to test interaction effects were formed using the centered predictor (Cohen, Cohen, West, & Aiken, 2003).

RESULTS

Sociodemographic and Health Characteristics

Table 1 presents sociodemographic and health characteristics for the entire sample, and by ethnicity and gender. Overall, participants were in their mid-twenties and single. Slightly over half of the participants described themselves as students. About one-quarter of participants had completed a college degree, and slightly less than three-quarters endorsed an annual household income at or below $40,000.00. Most participants were non-smokers, but frequent caffeine drinkers, and body mass index indicated that participants were overweight on average.

For age, and for body mass index, 2(Gender) × 2(Ethnicity) analysis of variance (ANOVA) was used to evaluate group differences. For age, a significant effect of ethnicity revealed that African American participants ($M = 25.55$ years, $SD = 5.64$) were an average of 2.27 years older than European American participants ($M = 23.28$ years, $SD = 4.82$), $F(1, 104) = 4.92, p < .03$. For body mass index (BMI), there was a significant effect of ethnicity, $F(1, 104) = 5.02, p < .03$, along with a trend ($p < .08$) for an ethnicity × gender interaction. The BMI of African American participants ($M = 30.13$ kg/m^2, $SD = 8.34$) exceeded that of European American participants ($M = 26.95$ kg/m^2, $SD = 6.50$) but, as shown in Table 1, this was primarily due to the relatively greater BMI of African American women. For the remaining sociodemographic and health characteristics, gender and ethnicity effects were tested in separate

TABLE 1. Sociodemographic and Health Characteristics for the Total Sample and by Ethnicity and Gender

		African American		European American	
	Total Sample (*N* = 108)	Women (*n* = 22)	Men (*n* = 22)	Women (*n* = 32)	Men (*n* = 32)
Age (years)	24.2 (5.27)	25.73 (5.51)	25.36 (5.90)	23.66 (5.11)	22.91 (4.55)
Body mass index (kg/m^2)	28.25 (7.44)	32.05 (8.57)	28.22 (7.84)	26.31 (7.12)	27.59 (5.87)
Not married/partnered (%)	81	86	86	78	78
Occupational status (% student)	58	41	41	59	81
College degree (%)	26	23	18	41	19
Income < $40,000.00 / year (%)	72	84	79	62	70
Smoke cigarettes (%)	28	14	36	34	25
Daily/almost daily caffeine (%)	79	77	77	75	84
Hormonal contraceptives (%)	–	23	–	47	–

Note. Values presented are percentages (%) or means (standard deviations) for entire sample, and for each demographic sub-group. *N*s as noted, except for income (*N* = 100).

chi-square analyses due to low cell frequencies when these two factors were crossed. These analyses revealed no significant gender differences. For ethnicity, African American individuals were less likely than European American individuals to endorse current student status (41% versus 70%, $\chi(108) = 9.27$, $p < .003$) and there was a trend ($p < .08$) for hormonal contraceptive use to be more prevalent among European American women compared to African American women.

Interpersonal Mistreatment and Trait Hostility

The average interpersonal mistreatment score across the entire sample was 9.20 ($SD = 5.41$). Regarding the two mistreatment subscales, 30 participants (28% of the sample) reported no experiences of blatant threats and accusations, whereas only four participants reported no instances of subtle disrespect. Participants' scores on the two subscales were significantly and positively correlated, $r(108) = .61$, $p < .0001$. A 2(Gender) × 2(Ethnicity) ANOVA revealed that men reported significantly more frequent mistreatment ($M = 10.17$, $SD = 5.62$) than women ($M = 7.74$, $SD = 4.81$), $F(1, 104) = 7.77$, $p < .007$; separate ANOVAs confirmed that this gender main effect held for both mistreatment subscales (*ps* < .04).

The average trait hostility score across the entire sample was 12.49 ($SD = 4.57$). A 2(Gender) × 2(Ethnicity) ANOVA revealed that men endorsed significantly higher levels of trait hostility ($M = 13.50$, $SD = 4.29$) than women ($M = 11.48$, $SD = 4.67$), $F(1, 104) = 5.42$, $p < .03$.

In the overall sample, trait hostility was positively and significantly associated with mistreatment, $r(108) = .31$, $p < .001$. Hierarchical regression was used to evaluate the independent contribution of trait hostility to interpersonal mistreatment and to assess whether this contribution varied by gender and ethnicity. As shown in Table 2, both male gender and trait hostility made significant and independent contributions to reports of interpersonal mistreatment. There was also a trend for a gender × ethnicity × hostility interaction. Follow-up of this interaction revealed significant associations between hostility and mistreatment among African American men only ($B = .87$, $p < .002$).

Discussion Topics Ratings

Across all three discussion topics, the average strength of opinion was 5.74 ($SD = .78$). Hierarchical regression was used to assess whether average strength of opinion differed by gender, ethnicity, interpersonal

TABLE 2. Hierarchical Regression Predicting Interpersonal Mistreatment from Trait Hostility, Gender, and Ethnicity

Step	Variable	*B*	*pr*	*t(df)*	*p*
1	Trait Hostility (H)	.31	.32	2.76 (104)	.007
	Gender (G)	2.31	.22	2.30 (104)	.02
	Ethnicity (E)	−.62	.00	−.62 (104)	.54
2	G × H	.28	.10	1.24 (101)	.22
	E × H	−.19	.00	−.82 (101)	.41
	G × E	1.31	.00	.64 (101)	.53
3	G × E × H	−.87	.17	−1.93 (100)	.06

Note. *B* = unstandardized regression coefficient; *pr* = partial correlation coefficient. Steps are hierarchical, each adjusted for all variables in the preceding step(s). Model R^2 = .19, $p < .003$

mistreatment, or their interactions. A significant main effect for ethnicity, $t(104) = -2.61$, $B = -.39$, $p < .02$, indicated that average strength of opinion was lower among European American participants ($M = 5.58$, $SD = .69$) than among African American participants ($M = 5.98$, $SD = .86$).

State Affect

Following baseline, average intensity ratings for fear and anger were .97 ($SD = 1.42$) and .86 ($SD = 1.75$), respectively. Multilevel models, adjusted for trait hostility, revealed no significant associations with gender, ethnicity, interpersonal mistreatment, or their interactions.

For both fear and anger, post-baseline ratings were subtracted from the mean of the three post-discussion ratings to form change-scores. Average post-discussion intensity ratings were 0.75 ($SD = 1.16$) for fear and 0.87 ($SD = 1.37$) for anger, and average change-scores were −.22 ($SD = 1.35$) and .01 ($SD = 2.07$), respectively. Multilevel models examined whether gender, ethnicity, interpersonal mistreatment, or their interactions, were associated with affective responses to the social interactions; trait hostility was entered as a covariate. For anger change-scores, a significant main effect of interpersonal mistreatment revealed that frequency of mistreatment was positively associated with anger reactivity during the discussions, $t(92.8) = 2.21$, $B = .17$, $p < .03$.

Interpersonal Mistreatment and Cardiovascular Responses

Table 3 presents average resting levels, discussion levels, and change-scores for each of the three cardiovascular measures, by ethnicity and gender. For systolic and diastolic blood pressure, resting levels and change-scores were uncorrelated, $rs(108) = -.02$ and $-.09$, respectively, $ps > .34$, supporting separate examination of these two cardiovascular processes. For heart rate, a small negative association was apparent between levels and change-scores, $r(108) = -.24$, $p < .02$.

Cardiovascular resting levels. Multilevel modeling for HR resting levels revealed a significant main effect for gender, with women showing higher levels than men, $B = -3.86$, $t(58.6) = -2.14$, $p < .04$. For SBP resting levels, as shown in Table 4, there were significant main effects of gender and ethnicity, both of which were qualified by a significant gender × ethnicity × interpersonal mistreatment interaction. Similarly, for DBP resting levels, there was a significant gender × ethnicity × interpersonal mistreatment interaction.

To follow-up these three-way interactions, we generated the simple slopes for the regression of interpersonal mistreatment on blood pressure for each of the four demographic sub-groups and then tested whether the simple slopes for the subgroups each differed from zero (Aiken & West, 1991). To illustrate the three-way interactions, we plotted the relationship between blood pressure resting levels and low (1 *SD* below the mean), average, and high (1 *SD* above the mean) levels of interpersonal mistreatment for each combination of gender and ethnicity. As illustrated in Figures 1 and 2, among African American men, frequency of self-reported interpersonal mistreatment was significantly and positively associated with both SBP, $B = .85$, $t(99) = 2.24$, $p < .03$, and DBP resting levels, $B = .59$, $t(97.9) = 2.23$, $p < .03$. In addition, as shown in Figure 1, interpersonal mistreatment was significantly and positively associated with SBP resting levels among European American women, $B = 1.17$, $t(98.9) = 2.39$, $p < .02$.

Cardiovascular reactivity. Multilevel modeling for cardiovascular change-scores revealed no significant effects for either HR or SBP. In contrast, as shown in Table 4, there was a trend ($p = .06$) for greater DBP reactivity among European American participants than African American participants. In addition, there was a significant gender × interpersonal mistreatment interaction. Examination of the simple slopes revealed a significant, positive association between interpersonal mistreatment and DBP reactivity for women, $B = .24$, $t(97.8) = 2.07$, $p = 0.04$, but a

TABLE 3. Cardiovascular Measures for the Total Sample and by Ethnicity and Gender

			African American		European American	
		Total Sample (N = 108)	Women (n = 22)	Men (n = 22)	Women (n = 32)	Men (n = 32)
SBP (mm/Hg)	Resting Level	114.52 (13.18)	112.19 (11.17)	124.22 (12.48)	105.53 (11.21)	118.45 (10.67)
	Discussion Level	122.66 (14.72)	119.67 (13.34)	131.70 (13.73)	113.06 (13.34)	128.08 (11.49)
	Change-Score	8.04 (6.68)	7.22 (7.47)	7.10 (7.10)	7.68 (6.91)	9.63 (5.52)
DBP (mm/Hg)	Resting Level	68.06 (7.97)	69.07 (8.62)	70.44 (7.80)	65.32 (7.18)	68.46 (7.98)
	Discussion Level	75.47 (8.66)	76.08 (9.61)	76.69 (8.07)	72.74 (8.22)	76.92 (8.55)
	Change-Score	7.38 (4.24)	6.99 (4.77)	6.03 (4.26)	7.50 (4.35)	8.47 (3.57)
HR (bpm)	Resting Level	69.47 (8.97)	71.67 (7.18)	67.29 (10.51)	70.52 (9.61)	68.39 (8.16)
	Discussion Level	74.69 (8.95)	77.74 (7.71)	70.55 (8.61)	76.52 (8.90)	73.61 (9.14)
	Change-Score	5.30 (4.17)	6.11 (4.80)	3.39 (4.58)	6.12 (3.87)	5.22 (3.39)

Note. SBP = systolic blood pressure; DBP = diastolic blood pressure; HR = heart rate. Values are averages, aggregated across all resting or discussion phases.

TABLE 4. Multilevel Modeling Results for Cardiovascular Resting Levels and Reactivity

		SBP Levels		DBP Levels		DBP Reactivity	
Step	Variable	*B*	*t(df)*	*B*	*t(df)*	*B*	*t(df)*
1	Trait Hostility	−.22	−.84 (90.5)	−.26	−1.45 (95.9)	−.10	−1.11 (74.1)
	Gender (G)	11.90	5.47** (58.1)	2.50	1.74 (59)	.26	.28 (58)
	Ethnicity (E)	6.08	2.62* (50.9)	2.98	1.77 (52)	−.14	−1.93 (50.9)
	Interpersonal Mistreatment (I)	.37	1.71 (99.4)	.15	1.00 (102)	.04	.52 (83.6)
2	G × E	−.31	4.51	−2.35	−.81 (55.5)	−1.31	−.70 (54.4)
	G × I	.19	.43	.34	1.19 (87.5)	−.39	−2.49 * (99.5)
	E × I	−.17	−.04 (98.4)	.14	.49 (100)	−.07	−.46 (84.4)
3	G × E × I	2.39	2.85 ** (94.5)	1.13	1.97* (88.5)	−.22	−.70 (98)

Note. SBP = systolic blood pressure; DBP = diastolic blood pressure; *B* = unstandardized regression coefficient. Steps are hierarchical, each adjusted for all variables in the preceding step(s). Variations in degrees of freedom between equivalent steps for SBP levels, DBP levels, and DBP reactivity are due to use of Satterthwaite's approximation.
$^{*}p \leq .05$; $^{**}p < .006$.

FIGURE 1. Predicted SBP resting level as a function of gender, ethnicity and low (*M*–1 *SD*), average (*M*), high (*M*+1 *SD*) levels of interpersonal mistreatment.

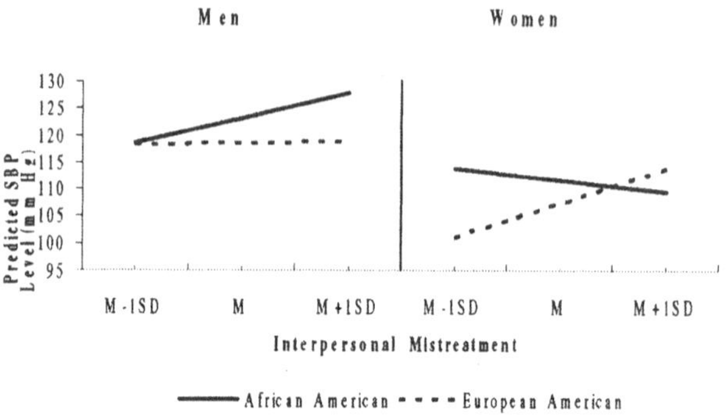

FIGURE 2. Predicted DBP resting level as a function of gender, ethnicity and low (*M*–1 *SD*), average (*M*), high (*M*+1 *SD*) levels of interpersonal mistreatment.

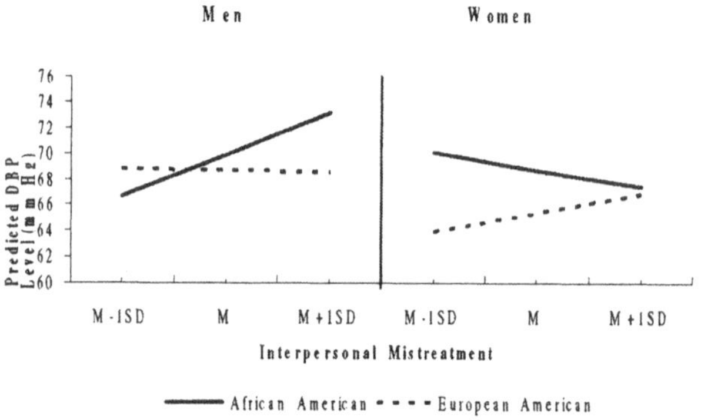

non-significant association for men, $B = -.13$, $t(97.6) = -1.31$, $p = .19$.[1]

DISCUSSION

The present study assessed associations between self-reported experiences of interpersonal mistreatment and cardiovascular responses measured in the context of problem-solving focused discussions with an opposite-gender partner. We evaluated cardiovascular resting levels and reactivity, two response patterns that have been identified as potential mediators between stressful experiences, including those of a social nature, and long-term health problems (McEwen, 1998). Broadly speaking, the results provide support for the hypothesized associations. Mistreatment was associated with elevated resting blood pressure levels and heightened blood pressure reactivity during brief problem-solving focused discussions, and some limited evidence for the predicted pattern of gender differences was observed. Furthermore, these associations were apparent after partialling variance due to trait hostility. Thus, despite its positive associations with trait hostility, particularly among African American men, interpersonal mistreatment emerged as an independent correlate of cardiovascular functioning. At the same time, some associations between mistreatment and blood pressure were moderated by gender and ethnicity in ways that were not predicted.

In support of our first hypothesis, we observed positive and significant associations between frequency of interpersonal mistreatment and resting systolic and diastolic blood pressure levels. These associations were apparent among African American men and European American women, but only for systolic blood pressure among the latter group of participants. One plausible explanation for these associations is that they reflect long-term consequences of exposure to relational adversity. For example, from roughly 22 to 32 years of age, emergence of blood pressure elevations is accelerated among individuals who show heightened reactivity to acute psychological stressors, such as that which has been shown to accompany direct exposure to adverse social experiences (Light et al., 1999). Moreover, this acceleration is particularly salient among individuals with a family history of hypertension, such as participants in the present study, who also endorse high levels of life stress. Thus, the elevated resting blood pressure we observed may reflect as individuals with a known vulnerability to hypertension. This does not, however, explain the specificity of these associations for African American men and European American women, indicating that other factors require consideration.

Psychosocial processes activated during the dyadic discussions, along with proximal features of the social setting, may have also contributed to resting blood pressure elevations. Although we designated cardiovascular levels "resting" levels, it seems probable that they reflect psychological processes that precede and follow stressful social interactions, such as anticipatory vigilance for social threat, or lingering anger that slows physiological recovery, rather than true "resting" levels marked by the absence of socioemotional activation (Glynn, Christenfeld, & Gerin,

2002; Smith, Ruiz, & Uchino, 2000). In this regard, the opposite-gender composition of the dyads deserves consideration. By increasing the salience of gender, opposite-gender social situations heighten accessibility of gender-related beliefs, many of which involve perceived differentials in status and hierarchical power (Ridgeway & Correll, 2004). Further, some evidence suggests that these perceived differentials vary by ethnicity. For example, among European American individuals as a whole, women are routinely presumed to possess less power and status than men (Ridgeway & Correll, 2004). In contrast, among African American individuals, some studies indicate that women are presumed to possess greater competence and status than men (Ridgeway & Correll, 2004), although there is more variability in such gender differentiation among African American compared to European American individuals (Filardo, 1996; Peters, Kinsey, & Malloy, 2004). Speculatively, the pattern of resting blood pressure elevations may reflect anticipation of, and lingering reactions to, interacting with a presumed more powerful individual, a process likely to be particularly salient among participants with histories of frequent mistreatment involving disrespect and experiences that affront social worth and rank.

In addition to associations with resting levels, frequent interpersonal mistreatment was also associated with elevations in diastolic blood pressure reactivity as individuals engaged in the discussions. This association was apparent among women only, despite the fact that men reported more frequent mistreatment than women, and even though frequent mistreatment was associated with elevated anger reactivity among men and women. This gender difference is generally consistent with the broader empirical literature on relational adversity, which has observed stronger linkages between negative aspects of social relationships and physiological reactivity for women than for men, although most of the relevant literature pertains to close relationships (e.g., Ewart et al., 1991). In the present study, it is important to consider these results in the context of the opposite-gender social interaction. That is, heightened DBP reactivity among women who have experienced frequent mistreatment may partially reflect the consequences of social interactions in which gender, and associated beliefs about power and status differentials, are highly salient.

The results of the present study, and particularly the unexpected patterns for gender and ethnicity, should be interpreted in light of a number of limitations. First, it is possible that some of the discussion topics may have revivified prior personal injustices, thereby activating memories and associated emotional and physiological responses among individuals with histories of mistreatment. Because we did not control for this, it is possible that only some, rather than all, participants were exposed to such topics. Further, if this exposure happened to vary by gender or ethnicity, this may have contributed to the pattern of interaction effects we observed. Future studies should explicitly control and compare the effects of stressors that are, and are not, reminiscent of mistreatment, as this process may be key to understanding how mistreatment experiences carry over to affect reactions to subsequent situations.

Second, we utilized a specific type of social interaction–a dyadic problem-solving task in which participants discussed current social issues about which they held at least moderately strong opinions. Thus, rather than standardizing topics, we allowed participants to choose topics of personal meaning to them. While some discussion topics (e.g., pollution) would not necessarily be associated with highly polarized opinions, other topics (e.g., smokers' rights) could be. Participants were not instructed to argue pro and con positions, but were to work together to arrive at mutually agreeable solutions. Nonetheless, pre-existing differences or similarities between interaction partners' opinions may have affected the socioemotional qualities of the discussions. Because we did not assess these similarities or differences, we were unable to evaluate whether or how they may have contributed to the pattern of results.

More generally, the results of the present study cannot be safely generalized to social settings in which gender is not a salient feature. Opposite-gender dyadic interactions activate a variety of specific gender-related belief systems and, as discussed above, some of these may be particularly activating to individuals with histories of frequent mistreatment. Thus, the specific pattern of results reported here could be a product of interpersonal mistreatment in combination with proximal features of the specific social setting, particularly gender-related features. Nonetheless, it is worth noting that opposite-gender social interactions occur commonly across multiple life domains, thereby offering a degree of ecological validity to the results of the present study (Ridgeway & Correll, 2004). In addition, this was a cross-sectional investigation. Although our implicit conceptual model is that interpersonal mistreatment leads to changes in cardiovascular response patterns, it is also plausible that pre-existing differences in physiological response systems lead to qualitatively different interpersonal experiences, or to qualitatively different emotional reactions upon exposure to mistreatment, thereby making the experiences more memorable and more likely to be reported on questionnaires. Only longitudinal investigations can begin to disentangle these possibilities. Finally, by selecting individuals who endorsed a parental history of hypertension, we studied a sample at elevated risk for future development of cardiovascular diseases (Burke et al., 1991). While it is unknown whether similar results will be observed among individuals not characterized by this vulnerability, research from animal models reveals that social stress contributes to cardiovascular pathology in the absence of predispositions to such problems (Andrews, Jenkins, Seachrist, Dunphy, & Ely, 2003).

The present results should also be considered within the context of the particular measure of interpersonal mistreatment that we administered. This measure taps exposure to hostile, threatening social interactions, and to situations that communicate disrespect and that affront one's social worth or rank. Selected because of its predictive validity with regard to important cardiovascular health outcomes in women, this measure developed out of the ethnic discrimination and racism literatures and was designed to capture commonplace interpersonal indignities (Williams et al., 1997). Despite these origins, in our study, the overall experiences of mistreatment that comprise this measure were equally common among European American and African American participants. Other studies have shown differences by ethnicity, but some show greater endorsement by African American individuals (Williams et al., 1997), whereas others show greater endorsement by European American individuals (Matthews, Salomon, Kenyon, & Zhou, 2005). Thus, when considering results across studies as a whole, this measure appears to tap mistreatment that is experienced by people broadly, with one exception: men endorsed more frequent mistreatment than women. Although we were initially surprised by this gender difference, it is identical to patterns observed by others that have employed the same measure of mistreatment (Kessler, Mickelson, & Williams, 1999; Matthews et al., 2005). Further, men's higher trait hostility levels did not account for this gender difference; both trait hostility and male gender made significant and unique contributions to reports of mistreatment, although this was most pronounced among African American men. While it may be that men experience more interpersonal mistreatment than women, it may also be that women discount instances of mistreatment, or that the measure we used does not tap experiences of mistreatment that are most common among women.

An additional feature of the measure of interpersonal mistreatment used here is that it is silent with respect to the source of mistreatment. Thus, we do not know if respondents used this measure to describe mistreatment experienced within relationships generally, or that experienced within close, intimate relationships, or both. Similarly, this measure does not differentiate ongoing mistreatment from mistreatment that has ended or has been resolved (Gump & Matthews, 1999). Both of these factors will be important to assess in future studies in order to develop a more refined understanding of connections between relational adversity and cardiovascular psychophysiology. More generally, there is a clear need for a conceptual mapping of relational adversity and interpersonal mistreatment, which could then be used to develop more comprehensive measures (Rook, 1998). Conceptualizations of interpersonal and psychological maltreatment, such as those emerging in literatures on emotional and psychological abuse in children (Glaser, 2002) and within close adult relationships (Follingstad & DeHart, 2000), may be helpful in this regard.

In sum, although not all hypotheses received consistent support, and some of the observed patterns were unexpected, the results of the present study illustrate associations between interpersonal mistreatment and blood pressure levels and reactivity. Both response patterns have been hypothesized to partially mediate connections between chronic stressors and long term negative health outcomes (McEwen, 1998). Considered along with documented associations between interpersonal mistreatment and objectively verified subclinical cardiovascular disease (Lewis et al., 2006; Troxel et al., 2003), this appears to be an area worthy of continued investigation. Future studies should examine processes that may mediate connections between mistreatment and blood pressure responses to social interactions (e.g., revivifying prior mistreatment) and should continue to explore how and why gender and ethnicity may moderate these connections. Efforts directed toward conceptualization and measurement of interpersonal mistreatment and related constructs will be essential to this endeavor.

NOTE

1. To examine whether the observed effects were stable across levels of condition (i.e., typical vs. maximal dominance), we re-ran all models including a main effect for condition, all two-way and three-way interactions involving condition, and the four-way interaction involving condition. In no case did condition moderate the effects reported in the present paper for either cardiovascular resting levels ($ps > .56$) or for reactivity ($p > .14$). However, there were three instances of significant effects involving condition (i.e., for resting SBP levels: condition × ethnicity × mistreatment; for resting HR levels: condition × gender × mistreatment; and for HR change-scores: condition × gender × ethnicity × interpersonal mistreatment). In the absence of hypotheses about

condition, we chose not to explore or interpret these interactions. However, future investigations might wish to consider how the specific socioemotional context affects individuals with histories of interpersonal mistreatment.

REFERENCES

Aiken, L. S., & West, S. G. (1991). *Multiple regression: Testing and interpreting interactions*. Newbury Park, CA: Sage.

Andrews, E., Jenkins, C., Seachrist, D., Dunphy, G., & Ely, D. (2003). Social stress increases blood pressure and cardiovascular pathology in a normotensive rat model. *Clinical and Experimental Hypertension, 25*, 85-101.

Barefoot, J. C., Dahlstrom, W. G., & Williams, R. B. (1983). Hostility, CHD incidence, and total mortality: A 25-year follow-up study of 255 physicians. *Psychosomatic Medicine, 45*, 59-63.

Barefoot, J. C., Dodge, K. A., Peterson, B. L., Dahlstrom, W. G., & Williams Jr., R. B. (1989). The Cook-Medley hostility scale: Item content and ability to predict survival. *Psychosomatic Medicine, 51*, 46-57.

Bloor, L. E., Uchino, B. N., Hicks, A., & Smith, T. W. (2004). Social relationships and physiological function: The effects of recalling social relationships on cardiovascular reactivity. *Annals of Behavioral Medicine, 28*, 29-38.

Borow, K. M., & Newberger, J. W. (1982). Noninvasive estimation of central aortic pressure during the oscillometric method for analyzing systemic artery pulsatile blood flow: Comparative study of indirect systolic, diastolic, and mean brachial artery pressure with simultaneous direct ascending aortic pressure measurements. *American Heart Journal, 103*, 879-886.

Brown, P. C., Smith, T. W., & Benjamin, L. S. (1998). Perceptions of spouse dominance predict blood pressure reactivity during marital interactions. *Annals of Behavioral Medicine, 20*, 286-293.

Burke, G., Savage, P., Sprafka, J., Selby, J., Jacobs, D., Jr, Perkins, L., Roseman, J., Hughes, G., & Fabsitz, R. (1991). Relation of risk factor levels in young adulthood to parental history of disease. The CARDIA study. *Circulation, 84*, 1176-1187.

Campbell, L., & Kashy, D. A. (2002). Estimating actor, partner, and interaction effects for dyadic data using PROC MIXED and HLM: A user-friendly guide. *Personal Relationships, 9*, 327-342.

Cohen, J., Cohen, P., West, S. G., & Aiken, L. S. (2003). *Applied multiple regression/correlation analysis for the behavioral sciences* (3rd ed.). Mahwah, N.J.: Lawrence Erlbaum.

Cook, W. W., & Medley, D. M. (1954). Proposed hostility and pharisaic-virtue scales for the MMPI. *Journal of Applied Psychology, 38*, 414-418.

Epstein, S. (1984). The stability of behavior across time and situations. In R. A. Zucker, J. Aronoff & A. I. Rabin (Eds.), *Personality and the Prediction of Behavior* (pp. 209-268). Orlando, FL: Academic.

Ewart, C. K., Taylor, C. B., Kraemer, H. C., & Agras, W. S. (1991). High blood pressure and marital discord: Not being nasty matters more than being nice. *Health Psychology, 10*, 155-163.

Filardo, E. K. (1996). Gender patterns in African American and White adolescents' social interactions in same-race, mixed-gender groups. *Journal of Personality and Social Psychology, 71*, 71-82.

Follingstad, D. R., & DeHart, D. D. (2000). Defining psychological abuse of husbands towards wives: Contexts, behaviors, and typologies. *Journal of Interpersonal Violence, 15*, 891-920.

Glaser, D. (2002). Emotional abuse and neglect (psychological maltreatment): A conceptual framework. *Child Abuse and Neglect, 26*, 697-714.

Glynn, L. M., Christenfeld, N., & Gerin, W. (2002). The role of rumination in recovery from reactivity: Cardiovascular consequences of emotional states. *Psychosomatic Medicine, 64*, 714-726.

Gump, B. B., & Matthews, K. A. (1999). Do background stressors influence reactivity to and recovery from acute stressors? *Journal of Applied Social Psychology, 29*, 469-494.

Guyll, M., Matthews, K. A., & Bromberger, J. T. (2001). Discrimination and unfair treatment: Relationship to cardiovascular reactivity among African American and European American women. *Health Psychology, 20*, 315-325.

Kamarck, T. W. (1992). Recent developments in cardiovascular reactivity: Contributions from psychometric theory and social psychology. *Psychophysiology, 29*, 491-503.

Kamarck, T. W., Annunziato, B., & Amateau, L. M. (1995). Affiliation moderates the effects of social threat on stress-related cardiovascular responses: Boundary conditions for a laboratory model of social support. *Psychosomatic Medicine, 57*, 183-194.

Kessler, R. C., Mickelson, K. D., & Williams, D. R. (1999). The prevalence, distribution, and mental health correlates of perceived discrimination in the United States. *Journal of Health and Social Behavior, 40*, 208-230.

Lepore, S. J., Mata, K. A., & Evans, G. W. (1993). Social support lowers cardiovascular reactivity to an acute stressor. *Psychosomatic Medicine, 55*, 518-524.

Lewis, T. T., Everson-Rose, S. A., Powell, L. H., Matthews, K. A., Brown, C., Karavolos, K. et al. (2006). Chronic exposure to everyday discrimination and coronary artery calcification in African American women: The SWAN Heart Study. *Psychosomatic Medicine, 68*, 362-368.

Light, K. C., Girdler, S. S., Sherwood, A., Bragdon, E. E., Brownley, K. A., West, S. G., & Hinderliter, A. L. (1999). High stress responsivity predicts later blood pressure only in combination with positive family history and high life stress. *Hypertension, 33*, 1458-1464.

Lovallo, W. R. (2005). Cardiovascular reactivity: Mechanisms and pathways to cardiovascular disease. *International Journal of Psychophysiology, 58*, 119-132.

Matthews, K. A., Salomon, K., Kenyon, K., & Zhou, F. (2005). Unfair treatment, discrimination, and ambulatory blood pressure in black and white adolescents. *Health Psychology, 24*, 258-265.

McEwen, B. S. (1998). Protective and damaging effects of stress mediators. *Seminars in Medicine of the Beth Israel Deaconess Medical Center, 338*, 171-179.

Murali, R., & Chen, E. (2005). Exposure to violence and cardiovascular and neuroendocrine measures in adolescents. *Annals of Behavioral Medicine, 30*, 155-163.

Newton, T. L., & Bane, C. M. H. (2001). Cardiovascular correlates of behavioral dominance and hostility during dyadic interaction. *International Journal of Psychophysiology, 40*, 33-46.

Newton, T. L., Parker, B. C., & Ho, I. K. (2005). Ambulatory cardiovascular functioning in healthy postmenopausal women with victimization histories. *Biological Psychology, 70*, 121-130.

Newton, T. L., & Sanford, J. M. (2003). Conflict structure moderates associations between cardiovascular reactivity and negative marital interaction. *Health Psychology, 22*, 270-278.

Peters, S., Kinsey, P., & Malloy, T. E. (2004). Gender and leadership perceptions among African Americans. *Basic and Applied Social Psychology, 26*, 93-101.

Pickering, T. G., & Kario, K. (2001). Nocturnal non-dipping: What does it augur? *Current Opinion in Nephrology and Hypertension, 10*, 611-616.

Ridgeway, C. L., & Correll, S. J. (2004). Unpacking the gender system: A theoretical perspective on gender beliefs and social relations. *Gender and Society, 18*, 510-531.

Rook, K. S. (1998). Investigating the positive and negative sides of personal relationships: Through a lens darkly? In B. H. Spitzberg & W. R. Cupach (Eds.), *The Dark Side of Close Relationships* (pp. 369-393). Mahwah, NJ: Lawrence Erlbaum Associates.

Seeman, T. E., & McEwen, B. S. (1996). Impact of social environment characteristics on neuroendocrine regulation. *Psychosomatic Medicine, 58*, 459-471.

Seeman, T. E., Singer, B. H., Ryff, C. D., Love, G. D., & Levy-Storms, L. (2002). Social relationships, gender, and allostatic load across two age groups. *Psychosomatic Medicine, 64*, 395-406.

Smith, T. W., Ruiz, J. M., & Uchino, B. N. (2000). Vigilance, active coping, and cardiovascular reactivity during social interaction in young men. *Health Psychology, 19*, 382-392.

Sterling, P., & Eyer, J. (1988). Allostasis: A new paradigm to explain arousal pathology. In S. Fisher & J. Reason (Eds.), *Handbook of Life Stress, Cognition and Health* (pp. 629-649). New York: John Wiley & Sons.

Suls, J., & Wan, C. K. (1993). The relationship between trait hostility and cardiovascular reactivity: A quantitative review and analysis. *Psychophysiology, 30*, 615-626.

Troxel, W. M., Matthews, K. A., Bromberger, J. T., & Sutton-Tyrrell, K. (2003). Chronic stress burden, discrimination, and subclinical carotid artery disease in African American and Caucasian women. *Health Psychology, 22*, 300-309.

Williams, D. R., Yu, Y., & Jackson, J. S. (1997). Racial differences in physical and mental health: Socio-economic status, stress, and discrimination. *Journal of Health Psychology, 2*, 335-351.

doi:10.1300/J135v07n02_03

Emotional Maltreatment and Verbal Victimization in Childhood: Relation to Adults' Depressive Cognitions and Symptoms

Brandon E. Gibb
Jessica S. Benas
Sarah E. Crossett
Dorothy J. Uhrlass

SUMMARY. Despite evidence that a history of childhood emotional maltreatment is related to the presence of a cognitive vulnerability to depression in adulthood, few studies have examined the relative impact of emotional maltreatment from parents versus verbal victimization from peers. In addition, no study of which we are aware has examined the relative impact of these forms of victimization on the presence of negative versus positive automatic thoughts in adulthood. Given this, we tested

---

Address correspondence to: Brandon E. Gibb, PhD, Department of Psychology, Binghamton University (SUNY), Binghamton, NY 13902-6000 (E-mail: bgibb@binghamton.edu).

This project was supported in part by National Institute of Mental Health grant MH 64301 and National Institute of Child Health and Human Development grant HD048664 awarded to the first author.

[Haworth co-indexing entry note]: "Emotional Maltreatment and Verbal Victimization in Childhood: Relation to Adults' Depressive Cognitions and Symptoms." Gibb, Brandon E. et al. Co-published simultaneously in *Journal of Emotional Abuse* (The Haworth Maltreatment & Trauma Press, an imprint of The Haworth Press, Inc.) Vol. 7, No. 2, 2007, pp. 59-73; and: *Childhood Emotional Abuse: Mediating and Moderating Processes Affecting Long-Term Impact* (ed: Margaret O'Dougherty Wright) The Haworth Maltreatment & Trauma Press, an imprint of The Haworth Press, Inc., 2007, pp. 59-73. Single or multiple copies of this article are available for a fee from The Haworth Document Delivery Service [1-800-HAWORTH, 9:00 a.m. - 5:00 p.m. (EST). E-mail address: docdelivery@haworthpress.com].

Available online at http://jea.haworthpress.com

doi:10.1300/J135v07n02_04

the hypothesis that negative and positive automatic thoughts would mediate the link between childhood emotional maltreatment and verbal victimization and young adults' current depressive symptoms. This hypothesis was supported. In addition, both emotional maltreatment and verbal victimization were independently related to the presence of negative automatic thoughts and both were significantly more strongly related to levels of negative thoughts than positive thoughts. doi:10.1300/J135v07n02_04

KEYWORDS. Abuse, depression, automatic thoughts, cognitive vulnerability

INTRODUCTION

In his cognitive theory of depression, Beck (1987; Beck, Rush, Shaw, & Emery, 1979; Clark, Beck, & Alford, 1999) proposed that the presence of a maladaptive self-referent schema centering on themes of failure, rejection, or worthlessness contributes vulnerability to the development of depression following the occurrence of negative life events. Although considered relatively trait-like, these schema are hypothesized to remain latent until activated by schema-congruent negative life events. Once activated, depressive schema are hypothesized to give rise to negative automatic thoughts regarding one's self, world, and future (referred to as the negative cognitive triad), which then contribute to the development of depression. In contrast to the trait-like depressive schema, negative automatic thoughts are hypothesized to be relatively state-like cognitions, generated without the person's conscious awareness, that contribute to depressive reactions following negative events and then dissipate with the alleviation of the depressed mood. Supporting Beck's theory, studies have found that changes in negative automatic thoughts predict changes in depressive symptoms (Dozois, 2002; Furlong & Oei, 2002; Philpot & Bamburg, 1996) and that they mediate the relation between dysfunctional attitudes and depressive symptoms (Kwon & Oei, 1994, 2003). Researchers (Kwon & Oei, 1992) have also found that negative automatic thoughts mediate the relation between negative life events and symptoms of depression.

Although the majority of research has focused on levels of negative automatic thoughts, Beck has suggested that depression is characterized not only by increases in negative automatic thoughts, but also decreases in positive automatic thoughts (e.g., Clark et al., 1999). Supporting Beck's distinction, studies have suggested that negative and positive automatic thoughts represent related but distinct constructs rather than opposite ends of the same continuum (for a review, see Clark et al., 1999). In addition, there is evidence that both types of automatic thoughts are independently related to levels of depressive symptoms (Dozois, 2002), supporting the importance of examining both within the same study. This said, however, it appears that depression is more strongly related to increased levels of negative thoughts than decreased levels of positive thoughts (e.g., Ingram, Slater, Atkinson, & Scott, 1990; Lightsey, 1994).

Given evidence for the relation between both negative and positive automatic thoughts and depressive symptoms, it is important to examine potential developmental antecedents to these thoughts. There is a growing body of research supporting the link between a history of childhood maltreatment and adults' cognitive vulnerability to depression (for a review, see Gibb, 2002). For example, building upon Rose and Abramson's (1992) developmental model, studies have supported the hypothesis that childhood emotional maltreatment by parents and verbal victimization from peers are related to the presence of a cognitive vulnerability to depression in young adults (Gibb et al., 2001; Gibb, Abramson, & Alloy, 2004).[1] In addition, there is evidence that these cognitive styles mediate the link between reports of childhood emotional maltreatment and both symptoms and diagnoses of depression among young adults (Gibb et al., 2001; Gibb, Alloy, Abramson, & Marx, 2003). Finally, there is evidence that verbal victimization prospectively predicts changes in children's cognitive styles and that these cognitive styles mediate the link between reports of verbal victimization and changes in children's depressive symptoms (Gibb & Alloy, 2006; Gibb, Alloy, Walshaw, Comer, Chang, & Villari, 2006).

A limitation of this line of research, however, is that it has focused almost exclusively on the development of negative cognitive styles. In contrast, potential developmental antecedents of positive thoughts have received less empirical attention. Therefore, it is not clear whether a history of emotional maltreatment or verbal victimization is related specifically to an increase in negative automatic thoughts or to both an increase in negative thoughts and a decrease in positive thoughts. Another limitation of past research is that victimization from parents and peers is rarely considered together in the same study. Although there is some evidence that both may contribute to the development of a cognitive vulnerability to depression (cf. Gibb et al., 2004), the relative contributions of emotional maltreatment and verbal victimization to positive versus negative automatic thoughts has not been explored. This type of investigation could be an important initial step in determining the relative impact of childhood victimization from parents versus peers as well as whether there is any specificity in terms of their effects on negative versus positive automatic thoughts.

The primary goal of this study, therefore, was to examine the relations among reports of negative childhood experiences, negative and positive automatic thoughts, and depressive symptoms in a cross-sectional study of young adults. Consistent with the results of previous studies (e.g., Gibb et al., 2001, 2003, 2004), we predicted that reports of both childhood emotional maltreatment and verbal victimization from peers would be related to participants' automatic thoughts. Furthermore, we predicted that these thoughts would mediate the relations of childhood emotional maltreatment and verbal victimization with young adults' depressive symptoms. A secondary goal was to examine the relative specificity of emotional maltreatment and verbal victimization to negative versus positive automatic thoughts. We predicted that reports of both childhood emotional maltreatment and verbal victimization would be more strongly related to levels of negative automatic thoughts than to positive automatic thoughts.

METHOD

Participants

Two hundred twelve undergraduates (156 women and 56 men), recruited from introductory psychology classes, participated in the current study. Of these, 121(57.1%) were Caucasian, 51(24.1%) were African American, 21(9.9%) were Asian, 8 (3.8%) were Hispanic, and the remaining 11(5.1%) participants either were from other ethnic groups or did not report their ethnicity. The mean age of the participants was 18.79 years (SD = 1.42).

Measures

Emotional maltreatment. Participants' histories of childhood emotional maltreatment by parents were assessed using the Life

Experiences Questionnaire (LEQ; Gibb et al., 2001). The LEQ was modeled on Cicchetti's (1989) Child Maltreatment Interview, but is more comprehensive and specific with respect to the events it assesses. For each event listed in the LEQ, participants indicate if they experienced the event before age 15, the age of onset and offset for the event described, its frequency of occurrence, and who the perpetrator was. Consistent with the suggestions made by Brewin, Andrews, and Gotlib (1993), the LEQ assesses a broad range of specific events rather than asking individuals for global estimates of maltreatment and neglect. The emotional maltreatment subscale of the LEQ has demonstrated predictive validity for episodes of depression (Gibb et al., 2001). In addition, levels of specific maltreatment experiences endorsed on the LEQ are related to depressive symptoms and cognitions whether or not participants label those experiences as maltreatment, suggesting that the relations are not due simply to a recall bias (Gibb, Alloy, & Abramson, 2003). Forms of emotional maltreatment assessed included derogation, humiliation, rejection, extortion, and teasing. Examples of items from the emotional maltreatment subscale include, "Did any of your caretakers ever say they wished they were not parents or that you had never been born?" and "Did anyone ever try to get you to do what he/she wanted by threatening you or someone you loved with physical harm?" Histories of emotional maltreatment were determined by summing the number of different maltreatment experiences endorsed by participants as having been committed by their parents (i.e., biological, step, adoptive, or other primary caretakers). Levels of emotional maltreatment by parents (LEQ-EM) could range from 0-51, with higher scores indicating more maltreatment. In this study, the LEQ-EM subscale exhibited good internal consistency ($\alpha = .86$).

Verbal peer victimization. Responses to the LEQ were also used to calculate levels of verbal peer victimization occurring before age 15. Scores on the peer victimization variable (LEQ-VV) were calculated by summing the number of experiences endorsed on the LEQ as having been committed by either peers or boy/girlfriends. Aside from the few items referring specifically to the behavior of parents (which were removed), these were the same items used to calculate levels of emotional maltreatment by parents. The difference lies in the subjects' report of who the perpetrator of the victimization was rather than in the type of experiences endorsed. Scores on this variable had a possible range of 0-45, with higher scores indicating more verbal victimization from peers. This subscale exhibited good internal consistency ($\alpha = .81$).

Automatic thoughts. Participants' negative and positive automatic thoughts were assessed using the Automatic Thoughts Questionnaire-Revised (ATQ-R; Kendall, Howard, & Hays, 1989). The ATQ-R consists of 30 negative self-statements (ATQ-R-N) and 10 positive self-statements (ATQ-R-P). Scores on each subscale were created by summing the relevant items, with higher scores indicating more negative (ATQ-R-N) or positive (ATQ-R-P) thoughts. Studies have supported the reliability and validity of the ATQ-R (e.g., Kendall et al., 1989). In this study, the ATQ-R-N and ATQ-R-P subscales exhibited excellent internal consistency (αs = .97 and .92, respectively).

Depressive symptoms. The Beck Depression Inventory (BDI; Beck et al., 1979) was used to assess participants' levels of depressive symptoms. Total scores on the BDI range from 0 to 63, with higher scores indicating more severe levels of depressive symptoms. Numerous studies have established the validity and reliability of the BDI (Beck, Steer, & Garbin, 1988). In the current study, the BDI exhibited excellent internal consistency ($\alpha = .90$).

Procedure

Participants were recruited from introductory-level psychology classes and received course credit for their participation. Participants completed all questionnaires in groups ranging in size from approximately five to 20.

RESULTS

Preliminary analyses revealed that a number of the variables exhibited significant skew. These variables were transformed (e.g., square root) prior to further analysis to satisfy assumptions of normality. Correlations among each of the variables as well as their means and standard deviations are presented in Table 1. To facilitate comparisons with other studies, the means and standard deviations presented are those for the untransformed variables.

As can be seen in Table 1, all of the variables were significantly intercorrelated. Focusing on the absolute magnitude of the correlations, we found that LEQ-EM was significantly more strongly related to ATQ-R-N than to ATQ-R-P, $z = 3.14$, $p = .001$ (cf. Meng, Rosenthal, & Rubin, 1992). The same pattern was also observed for LEQ-VV, $z = 2.64$,

TABLE 1. Correlations and Descriptive Statistics for Study Variables

	1	2	3	4	*M*	*SD*	Range
1. LEQ-EM	–				2.91	4.11	0-22
2. LEQ-VV	.46***	–			2.08	2.91	0-16
3. ATQ-R-N	.40***	.31**	–		49.88	20.15	30-149
4. ATQ-R-P	–.22**	–.16*	–.60***	–	32.54	8.76	11-50
5. BDI	.36**	.28***	.72***	–.62***	6.80	7.33	0-47

Note. LEQ-EM = Life Experiences Questionnaire-Emotional Maltreatment subscale. LEQ-VV = Life Experiences Questionnaire-Verbal Victimization subscale. ATQ-N = Automatic Thoughts Questionnaire-Revised Negative subscale. ATQ-P = Automatic Thoughts Questionnaire-Revised Positive subscale. BDI = Beck Depression Inventory.

*$p < .05$. **$p < .01$. ***$p < .001$.

$p = .004$. Consistent with the findings of previous studies, scores on the ATQ-R-N were significantly more strongly related to BDI scores than were scores on the ATQ-R-P, $z = 2.54$, $p = .005$. Finally, there were no significant differences in the magnitudes of the correlations of LEQ-EM versus LEQ-VV with ATQ-R-N, $z = 1.29$, $p = .10$, ATQ-R-P, $z = 0.86$, $p = .20$, or BDI, $z = 1.21$, $p = .11$, scores.

Next, the mediation hypothesis was tested using path analysis in AMOS 5 (Arbuckle, 2003). We first tested a full mediation model in which negative and positive automatic thoughts fully mediated the link between both childhood emotional abuse and verbal victimization and participants' current depressive symptoms. This model provided a good fit to the data, χ^2 (2, $N = 212$) = 4.35, $p = .11$, CFI = .99, RMSEA = .08, SRMR = .02 (cf. Hu & Bentler, 1999). The relations specified in the full mediation model accounted for 18% of the variance in ATQ-R-N scores, 5% of the variance in ATQ-R-P scores, and 57% of the variance in BDI scores. As can be seen in Figure 1, all of the paths included in this model were significant, with the exception of the path linking childhood verbal victimization to positive automatic thoughts. Thus, statistically controlling for the overlap between LEQ-EM and LEQ-VV, victimization from both sources remained significantly related to ATQ-R-N, but only LEQ-EM was related to ATQ-R-P. In addition, the magnitudes of the relations of LEQ-EM and LEQ-VV with ATQ-R-N did not differ significantly, $z = 1.28$, $p = .10$, suggesting that both forms of victimization were equivalently related to ATQ-R-N. Similarly, both ATQ-R-N and ATQ-R-P were uniquely related to BDI scores, although the magnitude of the ATQ-R-N path was significantly larger than the path from ATQ-R-P

FIGURE 1. Full Mediation Model. LEQ-EM = Life Experiences Questionnaire-Emotional Maltreatment subscale. LEQ-VV = Life Experiences Questionnaire-Verbal Victimization subscale. ATQ-N = Automatic Thoughts Questionnaire-Negative. ATQ-P = Automatic Thoughts Questionnaire-Positive. BDI = Beck Depression Inventory
*$p < .05$. **$p < .01$

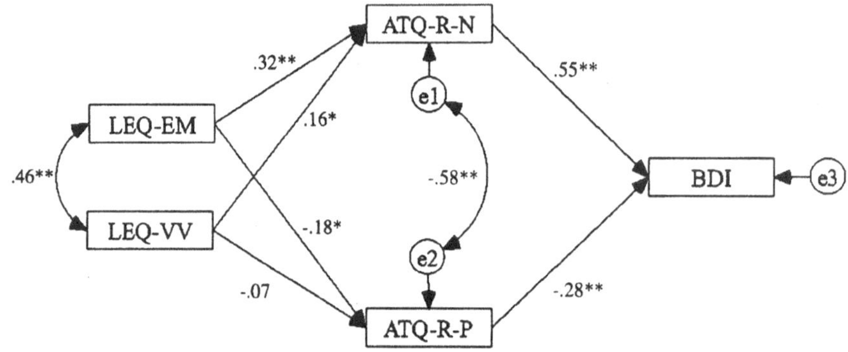

to BDI scores, $z = 9.77, p < .001$. Finally, although we also tested a partial mediation model, with direct paths added from LEQ-EM and LEQ-VV to BDI scores, neither of these additional paths were significant (both *ps* > .13), and this model did not fit significantly better than the more parsimonious full mediation model, $\chi^2(1, N = 212) = 4.35, p = .11$.

DISCUSSION

The purpose of the current study was to examine the relations among reports of negative childhood experiences, negative and positive automatic thoughts, and depressive symptoms in a cross-sectional study of young adults. Supporting our hypothesized mediational model, we found that negative and positive automatic thoughts fully mediated the link between childhood emotional maltreatment and verbal victimization and young adults' current depressive symptom levels. Supporting our specificity hypotheses, we found that victimization from both sources (caretakers and peers) was significantly more strongly related to negative than positive automatic thoughts. Further, although victimization from both sources was independently related to negative automatic thoughts, only childhood emotional maltreatment was related to positive thoughts, once the overlap between the two forms of victimization was statistically controlled. Finally, consistent with the findings of previous studies (e.g., Dozois, 2002; Ingram et al., 1990; Lightsey, 1994), we found that both negative and positive automatic thoughts were significantly related to depressive symptoms levels and that the magnitude of the relation was significantly stronger for negative thoughts.

The current results have potentially important implications for cognitive theories of depression (e.g., Clark et al., 1999; Rose & Abramson, 1992). Specifically, although cross-sectional, they are consistent with the growing body of research suggesting that both emotional maltreatment from parents and verbal victimization from peers may contribute to the development of negative cognitions and depressive symptoms (see also, Gibb et al., 2004; Gibb & Alloy, 2005; Gibb et al., 2001). Specifically, Rose and Abramson (1992) hypothesized that when negative events such as emotional maltreatment occur, children initially explain its occurrence in a way that will maintain their sense of hopefulness that it will not recur (e.g., "He was just in a bad mood today"). With repeated maltreatment, however, these hopefulness-maintaining explanations are repeatedly disconfirmed and the child may begin to make hopelessness-inducing explanations (e.g., "I can't do anything right"). With chronic and widespread maltreatment, these types of explanations would be hypothesized to develop into a trait-like depressive schema (e.g., "I'm worthless") that would then contribute to the expression of more state-like negative automatic thoughts following the occurrence of negative events. Although much of this hypothesized etiological model awaits empirical evaluation with longitudinal studies, there is evidence that experiences of verbal victimization do prospectively contribute to the development of children's cognitive vulnerability to depression (e.g., Gibb et al., 2006).

The current results also extend previous examinations of developmental correlates of depressive cognitions by suggesting that the negative effects of emotional maltreatment and verbal victimization may be relatively specific to the development of negative, as opposed to positive, thoughts. Thus, even though emotional maltreatment was significantly related to positive thoughts in our mediational model, the amount of variance accounted for was quite small. This is consistent with Rose and Abramson's (1992) model which, while not discussing positive thoughts specifically, did suggest that the development of negative cognitions would be more strongly tied to emotional maltreatment than other forms of negative events. This is expected because with emotional maltreatment the negative cognitions are directly supplied to the child by the abuser. To the extent that the content of emotional maltreatment and verbal victimization focuses on the presence of negative aspects about a child rather than the absence of positive aspects, these forms of victimization should be most strongly tied to the development of negative cognitions. Given that the current results are based upon a cross-sectional design, however, this hypothesis must remain tentative and should be explored more definitively in prospective longitudinal studies.

This said, however, participants' levels of positive thoughts were significantly related to reports of emotional maltreatment from parents, but not verbal victimization from peers. Therefore, it is possible that emotional maltreatment from parents, but not verbal victimization from peers, does affect the development of positive automatic thoughts. We may speculate about two possible reasons for this finding. First, it may be that individuals' positive self-statements are more strongly tied to messages received from parents than from other sources. A second possibility is that, because maltreatment from parents is likely to have an earlier age of onset than victimization from peers, that similar messages received from both sources have a greater effect upon one's positive thoughts at an earlier stage of development. In this view, one's positive thoughts–what has been referred to as the constructive schema (Clark et al., 1999)–may stabilize earlier in development than one's negative thoughts (depressive schema). Future longitudinal research with younger participants is needed to test this possibility.

The current results suggest a number of areas of future research. Most importantly, prospective longitudinal studies are needed to test the mediation model. Specifically, studies are needed to test the hypothesis that emotional maltreatment and verbal victimization actually contribute to the development of negative automatic thoughts and that these thoughts contribute risk to future depression. Given recent refinements in cognitive theories of depression (e.g., Hankin & Abramson, 2001), these studies should also examine potential transactional relations among victimization, negative thoughts, and depressive symptoms (cf. Gibb & Alloy, 2006). Specifically, it may be that early victimization sets in motion a vicious cycle of increasingly negative thoughts, depressive symptoms, and re-victimization. In addition, given evidence that different forms of maltreatment may have different effects based on the timing of their occurrence (e.g., Manly, Kim, Rogosch, & Cicchetti, 2001), combined with our finding that emotional maltreatment but not verbal victimization was related to participants' positive thoughts, future longitudinal studies should try to determine not only whether this result replicates, but also whether the key variable is the source of the victimization versus its timing. Finally, if the hypothesis that emotional maltreatment and verbal victimization contribute to the development of negative automatic thoughts is supported by future longitudinal studies, research will be needed to determine the stability of these thoughts once developed. That is, once developed, do automatic thoughts remain relatively stable like other forms of cognitive vulnerability to depression (e.g., negative attributional styles; see Gibb & Coles, 2005) and contribute chronic risk to depression over the lifespan? In addition to helping refine current theories of depression, the results of these future studies could have potentially important clinical implications for the development of more effective early intervention and prevention programs for at risk children, not only in terms of the suggested focus of these interventions, but also in terms of the most promising developmental time frame for their occurrence.

This study exhibited a number of strengths, including a strong foundation in theory regarding the nature and potential developmental antecedents of depressive symptoms, the assessment of childhood victimization from parents as well as peers, and the inclusion of reports of both positive and negative automatic thoughts. However, there were several limitations as well. First, as noted above, the study design was cross-sectional, and therefore no causal conclusions can be drawn. Prospective longitudinal studies with assessments beginning in childhood are needed to determine whether emotional maltreatment and verbal victimization are more likely to contribute to the actual development of negative versus positive thoughts. A second limitation was that all assessments were based on participants' self-report, which may have been subject to response or recall bias. That is, those who were currently depressed may have been more likely to remember and/or report instances of abuse in childhood than those who were not depressed. This said, however, studies have suggested that adults' recall of specific childhood events is relatively accurate (for a review, see Brewin et al., 1993). In addition, we have found that reports of emotional maltreatment assessed using the LEQ are significantly related to participants' cognitive styles, whether or not participants report believing that they were emotionally maltreated as a child, providing further support for the hypothesis that the results are not due simply to a recall bias (Gibb, Alloy et al., 2003). Despite this, future studies would benefit from assessments of maltreatment/victimization that do not rely upon participants' self-reports (e.g., observational methods or teacher reports). Finally, our sample consisted of undergraduate students with relatively low levels of depressive symptoms, which may limit our ability to generalize across populations. Future studies, therefore, should seek to replicate the current findings in other samples (e.g., psychiatric inpatients or outpatients, individuals with more severe histories of maltreatment, or more representative community samples of children drawn from public schools). This said, however, although this is the first study of which we are aware to examine the relations among emotional maltreatment from parents, verbal victimization from peers, negative and positive automatic thoughts, a number of studies have supported other links specified in our mediation model in more severely impaired samples. For example, there is support for the relation between a history of emotional maltreatment and diagnoses of depression in adult psychiatric outpatients (e.g., Gibb, Butler, & Beck, 2003; Gibb, Chelminski, & Zimmerman, 2007). In addition, the current results are consistent with previous studies in clinical samples (e.g., Kendall et al., 1989) suggesting that depression is more strongly linked to elevated levels of negative automatic thoughts than to lower levels of positive automatic thoughts. Based on these findings, we do have some confidence that our hypothesized mediational model will generalize to more impaired samples, though of course these individuals would be hypothesized to exhibit higher levels of victimization, negative automatic thoughts, and depression, and lower levels of positive automatic thoughts.

In summary, this study used a cross sectional design to examine the relations among reports of childhood emotional maltreatment from parents and verbal victimization from peers, and the presence of positive and negative automatic thoughts and depressive symptoms among young adults. In addition to finding support for the hypothesized mediational model, we found that victimization from both sources was independently related to negative thoughts and both were more strongly related to negative than positive automatic thoughts. These findings highlight the importance of examining victimization from both parents and peers in the development of cognitive vulnerability to depression and suggest that models proposed (e.g., Rose & Abramson, 1992) may be more applicable to the development of negative automatic thoughts than to positive thoughts. Future longitudinal studies are needed to more fully examine the extent to which emotional maltreatment and verbal victimization actually predict changes in negative automatic thoughts.

NOTE

1. It should be noted that both emotional maltreatment by parents and verbal peer victimization include the same behaviors (i.e., rejecting, humiliating, demeaning, and teasing). The key difference between these two forms of victimization lies in the child's relation to the perpetrator rather than in the type of behavior experienced.

REFERENCES

Arbuckle, J. L. (2003). *Amos 5* [Computer software]. Chicago: Smallwaters.

Beck, A. T. (1987). Cognitive models of depression. *Journal of Cognitive Psychotherapy, 1*, 5-37.

Beck, A. T., Rush, A. J., Shaw, B. F., & Emery, G. (1979). *Cognitive therapy of depression*. New York: Guilford.

Beck, A. T., Steer, R. A., & Garbin, M. G. (1988). Psychometric properties of the Beck Depression Inventory: Twenty-five years of evaluation. *Clinical Psychology Review, 8*, 77-100.

Brewin, C. R., Andrews, B., & Gotlib, I. H. (1993). Psychopathology and early experience: A reappraisal of retrospective reports. *Psychological Bulletin, 113*, 82-98.

Cicchetti, D. (1989). *Maltreatment Classification Interview*. Rochester, NY: University of Rochester, Mount Hope Family Center.

Clark, D. A., Beck, A. T., & Alford, B. A. (1999). *Scientific foundations of cognitive theory and therapy of depression*. New York: Wiley.

Dozois, D. J. A. (2002). Cognitive organization of self-schematic content in nondysphoric, mildly dysphoric, and moderately-severely dysphoric individuals. *Cognitive Therapy and Research, 26*, 417-429.

Furlong, M., & Oei, T. P. S. (2002). Changes to automatic thoughts and dysfunctional attitudes in group CBT for depression. *Behavioural and Cognitive Psychotherapy, 30*, 351-360.

Gibb, B. E. (2002). Childhood maltreatment and negative cognitive styles: A quantitative and qualitative review. *Clinical Psychology Review, 22*, 223-246.

Gibb, B. E., Abramson, L. Y., & Alloy, L. B. (2004). Emotional maltreatment by parents, verbal peer victimization, and cognitive vulnerability to depression. *Cognitive Therapy and Research, 28*, 1-21.

Gibb, B. E., & Alloy, L. B. (2006). A prospective test of the hopelessness theory of depression in children. *Journal of Clinical Child and Adolescent Psychology, 35*, 264-274.

Gibb, B. E., Alloy, L. B., & Abramson, L. Y. (2003). Global reports of childhood maltreatment versus recall of specific maltreatment experiences: Relationships with dysfunctional attitudes and depressive symptoms. *Cognition and Emotion, 17*, 903-915.

Gibb, B. E., Alloy, L. B., Abramson, L. Y., & Marx, B. P. (2003). Childhood maltreatment and maltreatment-specific inferences: A test of Rose and Abramson's (1992) extension of the hopelessness theory. *Cognition and Emotion, 17*, 917-931.

Gibb, B. E., Alloy, L. B., Abramson, L. Y., Rose, D. T., Whitehouse, W. G., Donovan, P., et al. (2001). History of childhood maltreatment, depressogenic cognitive style, and episodes of depression in adulthood. *Cognitive Therapy and Research, 25*, 425-446.

Gibb, B. E., Alloy, L. B., Walshaw, P. D., Comer, J. S., Chang, G. H., & Villari, A. G. (2006). Predictors of attributional style change in children. *Journal of Abnormal Child Psychology, 34*, 425-439.

Gibb, B. E., Butler, A. C., & Beck, J. S. (2003). Childhood abuse, depression, and anxiety in adult psychiatric outpatients. *Depression and Anxiety, 17*, 226-228.

Gibb, B. E., Chelminski, I., & Zimmerman, M. (2007). *Childhood emotional, physical, and sexual abuse and diagnoses of depressive and anxiety disorders in adult psychiatric outpatients. Depression and Anxiety, 24*, 256-263.

Gibb, B. E., & Coles, M. E. (2005). Cognitive vulnerability-stress models of psychopathology: A developmental perspective. In B. L. Hankin & J. R. Z. Abela (Eds.), *Development of psychopathology: A vulnerability-stress perspective* (pp. 104-135). Thousand Oaks, CA: Sage.

Hankin, B. L., & Abramson, L. Y. (2001). Development of gender differences in depression: An elaborated cognitive vulnerability-transactional stress theory. *Psychological Bulletin, 127*, 773-796.

Hu, L., & Bentler, P. M. (1999). Cutoff criteria for fit indexes in covariance structure analysis: Conventional criteria versus new alternatives. *Structural Equation Modeling, 6*, 1-55.

Ingram, R. E., Slater, M. A., Atkinson, J. H., & Scott, W. (1990). Positive automatic cognition in major affective disorder. *Psychological Assessment, 2*, 209-211.

Kendall, P. C., Howard, B. L., & Hays, R. C. (1989). Self-referent speech and psychopathology: The balance of positive and negative thinking. *Cognitive Therapy and Research, 13*, 583-598.

Kwon, S., & Oei, T. P. S. (1992). Differential causal roles of dysfunctional attitudes and automatic thoughts in depression. *Cognitive Therapy and Research, 16*, 309-328.

Kwon, S., & Oei, T. P. S. (1994). The roles of two levels of cognitions in the development, maintenance, and treatment of depression. *Clinical Psychology Review, 14*, 331-358.

Kwon, S., & Oei, T. P. S. (2003). Cognitive change processes in a group cognitive behavior therapy of depression. *Journal of Behavior Therapy and Experimental Psychiatry, 34*, 73-85.

Lightsey, O. R. (1994). Positive automatic cognitions as moderators of the negative life event-dysphoria relationship. *Cognitive Therapy and Research, 18*, 353-365.

Manly, J. T., Kim, J. E., Rogosch, F. A., & Cicchetti, D. (2001). Dimensions of child maltreatment and children's adjustment: Contributions of developmental timing and subtype. *Development and Psychopathology, 13*, 759-782.

Meng, X., Rosenthal, R., & Rubin, D. B. (1992). Comparing correlated correlation coefficients. *Psychological Bulletin, 111*, 172-175.

Philpot, V. D., & Bamburg, J. W. (1996). Rehearsal of positive self-statements and restructured negative self-statements to increase self-esteem and decrease depression. *Psychological Reports, 79*, 83-91.

Rose, D. T., & Abramson, L. Y. (1992). Developmental predictors of depressive cognitive style: Research and theory. In D. Cicchetti & S. Toth (Eds.), *Rochester symposium of developmental psychopathology, Vol. IV* (pp. 323-349). Rochester, NY: University of Rochester Press.

doi:10.1300/J135v07n02_04

The Impact of Childhood Psychological Abuse on Adult Interpersonal Conflict: The Role of Early Maladaptive Schemas and Patterns of Interpersonal Behavior

Terri L. Messman-Moore
Aubrey A. Coates

SUMMARY. The impact of childhood psychological abuse on adult interpersonal conflict was examined among 382 college women. Psychological abuse predicted adult interpersonal conflict above and beyond the effects of parenting behavior (i.e., parental warmth and control). The relationship between psychological abuse and conflict was mediated or partially mediated by three early maladaptive schemas: mistrust/abuse, abandonment,

---

Address correspondence to: Terri L. Messman-Moore, PhD, Department of Psychology, Miami University, 90 North Patterson Avenue, Oxford, OH 45056 (E-mail: messmat@muohio.edu).

The authors would like to acknowledge numerous research assistants, without whom this project would not be possible: Alicyndra Amundsen, Erin Bybee, Dasi Ginnis, Sarah Hoskinson, Julie Krizay, Erin Kupres, Jenni Oberlag, and Mai Foerster Shaffner.

An earlier version of this paper was presented at the annual meeting of the Advancement of Behavioral and Cognitive Therapies, November 2005, in Washington, DC.

[Haworth co-indexing entry note]: "The Impact of Childhood Psychological Abuse on Adult Interpersonal Conflict: The Role of Early Maladaptive Schemas and Patterns of Interpersonal Behavior." Messman-Moore, Terri L., and Aubrey A. Coates. Co-published simultaneously in *Journal of Emotional Abuse* (The Haworth Maltreatment & Trauma Press, an imprint of The Haworth Press. Inc.) Vol. 7, No. 2, 2007, pp. 75-92; and: *Childhood Emotional Abuse: Mediating and Moderating Processes Affecting Long-Term Impact* (ed: Margaret O'Dougherty Wright) The Haworth Maltreatment & Trauma Press, an imprint of The Haworth Press, Inc., 2007, pp. 75-92. Single or multiple copies of this article are available for a fee from The Haworth Document Delivery Service [1-800-HAWORTH, 9:00 a.m. - 5:00 p.m. (EST). E-mail address: docdelivery@haworthpress.com].

Available online at http://jea.haworthpress.com

doi:10.1300/J135v07n02_05

and defectiveness/shame. Paternal warmth had a significant, direct relationship with interpersonal conflict. The association between mistrust/abuse schemas and interpersonal conflict was partially mediated by three patterns of interpersonal behavior: overly accommodating behavior, social isolation, and domineering/controlling behavior. Of the three patterns, domineering/controlling behavior explained the most variance in adult conflict. Findings provide support for the long-lasting impact of childhood psychological abuse and suggest that effects of psychological abuse persist via early maladaptive schemas. doi:10.1300/J135v07n02_05

KEYWORDS. Child maltreatment, psychological abuse, early maladaptive schemas, interpersonal behavior

INTRODUCTION

Accepted parenting strategies often lie on the same continuum as psychologically abusive behavior. For example, giving a child a "time-out" is a well-accepted method of discipline for children. However, when the "time-out" is extended for long periods of time, such as days or weeks, it would most likely be considered abusive. Shouting at a child, calling a child names, or shaming a child are behaviors also used as disciplinary tactics (Straus & Field, 2003). The difficulty lies in deciding where on the continuum "normal" parenting behavior becomes abusive. Child maltreatment researchers have struggled to agree upon a precise, but comprehensive definition of psychological abuse (PA). Hart, Brassard, Bineggeli, and Davidson (2002) identified five types of behavior by the caregiver toward the child which may indicate psychological abuse: spurning (rejecting or degrading the child), terrorizing (threatening injury, death, or abandonment of the child, or of people or objects the child loves), isolating (refusing the child opportunities to interact with others), exploiting/corrupting (encouraging engagement in inappropriate behaviors), or denying emotional responsiveness (ignoring the child's needs for interaction and affection). Furthermore, they proposed a definition of PA which specifies that the abusive behavior of the caregiver is a repeated pattern or so severe as to communicate to the child that he or she is "worthless, flawed, unloved, unwanted, endangered, or only of value in meeting another's needs" (Hart et al., 2002, p. 81).

In a recent study of the prevalence of childhood maltreatment in a community sample of adults, the prevalence of childhood PA was approximately 14% for women and 10% for men, with between 3% and 8% of the total sample having experienced psychological abuse in conjunction with another type of maltreatment (Scher, Forde, McQuaid, & Stein, 2004). Research suggests that PA may have both immediate and long-lasting harmful effects. Among children, PA has been associated with depression (Kaufman, 1991), depressive attributional styles (Cerezo & Frias, 1994), delinquency, and interpersonal problems (Vissing, Straus, Gelles, & Harrop, 1991). These effects are not limited to childhood, however. Adults with a history of PA during childhood also report problems with depression, anxiety, interpersonal sensitivity (Briere & Runtz, 1988), emotional inhibition (Krause, Mendelson, & Lynch, 2003), low self-esteem (Briere & Runtz, 1990; Gross & Keller, 1992), suicidal behavior (Mullen, Martin, Anderson, Romans, & Herbison, 1996), somatic complaints, post-traumatic stress symptoms (Spertus, Yehuda, Wong, Halligan, & Seremetis, 2003), and difficulties with adult relationships (Varia & Abidin, 1999).

The study of PA is complicated given that "emotional maltreatment could be broadly conceptualized as a component of all forms of maltreatment, including sexual and physical abuse" (Bernstein, 2002, p. 618). Despite assumptions that other forms of child abuse (i.e., physical and sexual) often co-exist (Higgins & McCabe, 2001), less is known about whether PA occurs more frequently in isolation or in conjunction with other types of maltreatment. However, even when PA occurs alone, it appears to exert a significant impact on adult functioning. Clemmons (2005) found that college students reporting only PA had higher levels of psychological distress compared to individuals reporting only physical abuse or childhood neglect. Finally, the role of PA in adult functioning seems important even when it occurs with other forms of childhood abuse. McGee, Wolfe, and Wilson (1997) argue that psychological maltreatment often potentiates the effects of other types of child abuse (e.g., physical or sexual). Other studies indicate that PA predicts later maladaptive outcomes over and above other types of abuse (Claussen & Crittenden, 1991; Gross & Keller, 1992).

PSYCHOLOGICAL ABUSE AND EARLY MALADAPTIVE SCHEMAS

Although there is growing evidence for a link between childhood PA and poor adult functioning, less is known about the mechanisms underlying this relationship. Moran, Bifulco, Ball, Jacobs and Benaim (2002) suggest that childhood PA increases levels of shame, which impacts levels of depression and perhaps other forms of pathology. Another broader explanation is that PA in childhood impacts the developing understanding of self and others, which in turn impacts psychological functioning and interpersonal behavior. Young, Klosko, and Weishaar (2003) argue that formative childhood experiences contribute to early maladaptive schemas (EMS), rigid interpersonal beliefs that are dysfunctional and repeat throughout life. An early maladaptive schema is defined as a "broad, pervasive theme or pattern comprised of memories, emotions, cognitions, and bodily sensations regarding oneself and one's relationships with others . . . [that] are dysfunctional to a certain degree" (p. 7). PA would presumably contribute to EMS, which form the foundation for one's general view of self and others.

Children who experience PA may develop EMS along the theme of interpersonal disconnection and rejection. Schemas within this domain often have the most significant, long-lasting impact because these schemas interfere with one's ability to form secure, satisfying attachments to others. EMS that others are untrustworthy or will be abusive, that others will abandon or deprive the individual of emotional connection, or beliefs of shame and defectiveness may play an important role in poor interpersonal relatedness experienced during adulthood (Young et al., 2003). EMS are critical to current functioning because they drive information processing and interpretation of experience, filtering input which further strengthens these belief systems. At least one previous study has linked PA to several EMS, including mistrust and abuse, emotional deprivation, and defectiveness and shame schemas (Cecero, Nelson, & Gillie, 2004). Although hypothesized, PA was not associated with abandonment schemas. In that study, mistrust/abuse schemas were associated only with PA; there was no relationship between these schemas and other forms of child maltreatment such as sexual abuse, physical abuse or emotional neglect. However, the theory proposed by Young and colleagues (2003) presumes that any form of child maltreatment (or other negative, formative experience) would influence the formation of these schemas.

Although there is some preliminary evidence for a relation between PA and early maladaptive schemas, we cannot assume that EMS inevitably lead to maladaptive behavior. According to Young's theory, schemas impact behavior via three general coping styles: surrender, avoidance, and overcompensation (Young et al., 2003). Surrender involves "yielding" to a schema. Individuals do not try to avoid or fight the schema, and without awareness often repeat schema-driven patterns which, in the case of deprivation and rejection schemas, would result in passive, compliant, or subjugating adult behavior. Avoidance involves "fleeing" from the schema by avoiding persons or situations that may trigger these beliefs or a sense of vulnerability. An avoidant coping style may lead abused individuals to become socially inhibited or to avoid intimate relationships and other interpersonal situations that trigger the schema. Overcompensation involves "fighting" the schema by acting in opposition to the schema. Although resisting the schema can be healthy, overcompensation involves an extreme response seemingly out of proportion to the situation. This coping style may lead to behavior reminiscent of the perpetrator that is controlling, domineering, or callous. Thus, psychologically abused individuals may respond to the mistrust/abuse schema by surrendering to (e.g., subjugating oneself), avoiding (e.g., becoming socially inhibited), or overcompensating (e.g., dominating or controlling others) for the schema.

Few studies are available which examine the long-term impact of child PA, and even fewer focus on interpersonal functioning. Schema theory offers one framework to examine interpersonal effects and may be a particularly useful framework to understand the complex and diverse outcomes associated with child PA. First, children may or may not develop EMS in relation to PA. The absence of EMS may be a marker of resilience in cases where an adult who experienced child PA does not appear to suffer from negative long-term psychological or interpersonal consequences. Second, if abused children do develop a common belief (EMS) around mistrust and abuse, there may be differences in outward behavior and functioning as a result of coping style. Given this, schema theory helps to account for the heterogeneity of outcomes associated with abuse that sometimes appear incompatible (e.g., submissive versus controlling behavior in response to PA).

Aims of the Current Study

The current study aims to examine the relationship between childhood PA and adult interpersonal functioning. The first aim is to replicate and extend findings from earlier studies establishing a link between PA and problematic interpersonal functioning in adulthood (e.g., Varia & Abidin, 1999). Given that PA may lie on a continuum with normal parenting practices, we will also consider the impact of parenting (as measured by parental warmth and control) when examining the role of PA. The second aim of the current study is to use Young's schema theory (Young et al., 2003) as a framework to explain the long-term effects of PA. In particular, we propose that the relationship between PA and adult interpersonal conflict will be mediated by one or more early maladaptive schemas characteristic of disconnection and rejection (i.e., mistrust/abuse, abandonment, emotional deprivation, and defectiveness/shame). Finally, we propose that coping styles, in the form of interpersonal behavioral patterns, will mediate the relation between EMS and interpersonal conflict. Three coping styles will be examined: schema surrender (overly accommodating behavior), schema avoidance (socially inhibited behavior), and schema overcompensation (domineering and controlling behavior).

METHOD

Participants

Participants included 382 college women recruited from Introduction to Psychology courses for a study on "College Women's Beliefs about Interpersonal Relationships." Women were either students at the main campus of a midsized, Midwestern university or were students at a smaller, satellite campus of the same university. Participants ranged in age from 17-51 (mean age = 19.3, *SD* = 3.4). Most participants were Caucasian (92.4%). The majority were unmarried (87.1%), although 7.1% reported that they were married or living with a partner. The majority of participants' parents were well educated, with 68.9% of participants' fathers having received at least a college degree and 63.9% of participants' mothers having received at least a college degree. Most participants (57%) reported family incomes greater than $75,000.

Measures

Computer Assisted Maltreatment Inventory (CAMI). The CAMI (DiLillo, 2003; Nash, DiLillo, Messman-Moore & Rinkol, 2002) is a retrospective self-report measure of childhood stressors including physical abuse, sexual abuse, psychological abuse, neglect, and witnessing domestic violence. The Psychological Abuse (PA) scale includes 57 behaviorally specific questions designed to assess 5 domains of PA during childhood: emotional unresponsiveness, demandingness, terrorizing/spurning, isolating, and corrupting. For the current study, a total score was computed. Internal consistency alphas for the PA scale have ranged from .90 to .96 in college and community samples (Nash, 2005), and was .95 in the current study.

Parental Bonding Instrument (PBI). The PBI (Parker, Tupling, & Brown, 1979) is a 25-item retrospective self-report measure of respondents' perception of their caregiver's parenting style during their first 16 years. The PBI consists of two sub-scales: warmth/care and control/overprotection, which are calculated for both maternal and paternal caregivers. The PBI has demonstrated sufficient reliability and validity (Parker et al., 1979). Internal consistency alphas in the current study ranged from .81 to .95.

Young Schema Questionnaire–Short Form (YSQ-S). The YSQ-S (Young et al., 2003) is a 75-item self-report questionnaire that assesses Early Maladaptive Schemas (EMS). The short form is an abbreviated version of the full 205-item measure designed to measure 16 EMS. The current study focused on four EMS: Abandonment (AB), Emotional Deprivation (ED), Mistrust/Abuse (MA), and Defectiveness/Shame (DS). The primary subscales possess adequate internal consistency, with alphas ranging from .83 to .96 (Schmidt, Joiner, Young, & Telch, 1995). In the current study, internal consistency alphas ranged from .75 to .86.

Inventory of Interpersonal Problems (IIP). The IIP (Horowitz, Alden, Wiggins, & Pincus, 2000) is a 64-item self-report measure that assesses respondent's interpersonal difficulties. The current study focused on three of the seven subscales: domineering/controlling (DC), socially inhibited (SI), and overly accommodating (OA). A standardization sample revealed internal consistency alphas for the subscales to range from .76 to .85 (Horowitz et al., 2000). The current study found internal consistency alphas of .81 for DC, .85 for OA, and .89 for SI.

Inventory of Altered Self-Capacities (IASC). The IASC (Briere, 1998) is a 63-item self-report measure of difficulties in the areas of relationships, identity, and affect regulation. The Interpersonal Conflict (IC) subscale was used to examine the tendency to be involved in distressing relationships. Representative items include: "Having trouble getting along with people at work, school, or in your neighborhood," "Having lots of ups and downs in your relationships with people," and "Getting into arguments with people." Scales of the IASC, including IC, may be associated with borderline personality features. Briere (1998) reported that the IC scale had significantly higher correlations with the borderline features scale of the Personality Assessment Inventory, compared to the antisocial and paranoia scales. Internal consistency alphas for the IC subscale ranged from .88 to .90 for normative and university samples (Briere, 1998) and was .91 in the current study.

RESULTS

Data Analysis

All statistical analyses were conducted with SPSS 13.0 for Windows. Several sets of analyses were conducted to test the hypotheses. First, bivariate correlations were calculated to determine whether variables were associated as hypothesized and to determine whether the basic requirements were met to test for mediation (Baron & Kenny, 1986). Second, all four proposed mediators (mistrust/abuse, abandonment, defectiveness/shame, and emotional deprivation schemas) were examined together as predictors of interpersonal conflict. Based on the results of this linear regression analysis, additional sets of regression analyses were conducted, using the steps outlined by Baron and Kenny (1986) to determine whether schemas mediated the relationship between PA and interpersonal conflict. Another set of analyses was conducted to determine whether interpersonal behavior mediated the relation between EMS and interpersonal conflict.

General Associations

Bivariate correlations were calculated for all variables of interest (see Table 1). As hypothesized, childhood PA was positively correlated with parental control and negatively associated with parental warmth for both maternal and paternal caregivers. Given this relation, the four parenting variables were included in later analyses in which mediation was tested. Higher levels of PA were also positively correlated with higher levels of interpersonal conflict and greater endorsement of the early maladaptive schemas.

Predicting Interpersonal Conflict

In order to examine the relative importance of the four different schemas as predictors of interpersonal conflict, a stepwise linear regression analysis

TABLE 1. Bivariate Correlations

	PA	MW	PW	MC	PC	IC	ED	AB	MA	DS
PA	1									
MW	–.69**	1								
PW	–.60**	.38**	1							
MC	.45**	–.41**	–.26**	1						
PC	.44**	–.26**	–.36**	.42**	1					
IC	.36**	–.23**	–.31**	.20**	.14**	1				
ED	.41**	–.42**	–.30**	.16**	.16**	.34**	1			
AB	.41**	–.25**	–.22**	.15**	.17**	.39**	.37**	1		
MA	.37**	–.23**	–.23**	.19**	.18**	.49**	.37**	.51**	1	
DS	.25**	–.11*	–.18**	.07	.10	.35**	.37**	.27**	.43**	1

PA = Psychological Abuse (CAMI); MW = Maternal Warmth (PBI); PW = Paternal Warmth (PBI); MC = Maternal Control (PBI); PC = Paternal Control (PBI); IC = Interpersonal Conflict (IASC); ED = Emotional Deprivation (YSQ); AB = Abandonment (YSQ); MA = Mistrust/Abuse (YSQ); DS = Defectiveness/Shame (YSQ)
** Correlation is significant at the .01 level (2-tailed).
* Correlation is significant at the .05 level (2-tailed).

was conducted to examine the impact of PA (controlling for parental warmth and control) and four EMS (abandonment, mistrust/abuse, defectiveness/shame, and emotional deprivation) on interpersonal conflict. Stepwise procedures were utilized to examine the individual contribution of each set of variables. Maternal and paternal warmth and control were entered on the first step, PA was entered on the second step, and the four schemas were entered on the third step. The model was significant at each step (see Table 2). In the final model, there were four significant predictors: paternal warmth, abandonment schemas, mistrust/abuse schemas, and defectiveness/shame schemas, ANOVA $F(9,296) = 18.46, p < .001$. Emotional deprivation was not a significant predictor in the multivariate model. PA was not a significant predictor of interpersonal conflict when early maladaptive schemas were included in the model (Step 3). Because these results suggest that EMS may mediate the relation between PA and interpersonal conflict, additional analyses were conducted to specifically test for mediation.

Tests of Mediation: Schemas

The first set of analyses aimed to test whether EMS mediated the relation between child PA and adult interpersonal conflict. According to

TABLE 2. Predicting Interpersonal Conflict from Parenting Behavior, Psychological Abuse, and Early Maladaptive Schemas

	Variable	B	SE(B)	Beta	*t*	*p*	R^2	Adj R^2
Step 1						.001	.14	.12
	Maternal Warmth	–.11	.06	–.11	–1.82	.07		
	Paternal Warmth	**–.18**	**.05**	**–.24**	**–3.95**	**.001**		
	Maternal Control	.12	.06	.12	1.88	.06		
	Paternal Control	.00	.07	.00	.02	.98		
Step 2						.001	.17	.15
	Maternal Warmth	.03	.07	.03	.35	.72		
	Paternal Warmth	**–.12**	**.05**	**–.16**	**–2.35**	**.02**		
	Maternal Control	.08	.06	.08	1.31	.19		
	Paternal Control	–.04	.07	–.04	–.65	.52		
	Psychological Abuse	**.07**	**.02**	**.29**	**3.33**	**.001**		
Step 3						.001	.36	.34
	Maternal Warmth	.01	.07	.01	.17	.87		
	Paternal Warmth	**–.10**	**.04**	**–.14**	**–2.34**	**.02**		
	Maternal Control	.08	.06	.08	1.50	.13		
	Paternal Control	–.06	.06	–.05	–.92	.36		
	Psychological Abuse	.01	.02	.06	.75	.45		
	Emotional Deprivation	.33	.42	.05	.80	.43		
	Abandonment	**.70**	**.35**	**.12**	**1.99**	**.05**		
	Mistrust/Abuse	**1.56**	**.32**	**.30**	**4.93**	**.001**		
	Defectiveness/Shame	**1.95**	**.63**	**.17**	**3.08**	**.002**		

Baron and Kenny (1986), several assumptions must be met for mediation to be present. First, the independent variable (i.e., PA) must predict the dependent variable (i.e., interpersonal conflict). Second, the independent variable must predict the mediator (i.e., early maladaptive schemas). Third, the mediator must predict the dependent variable. Finally, the impact of the independent variable on the dependent variable must be reduced or become nonsignificant when the mediator is included in the equation. To fulfill these requirements, three sets of analyses were conducted, one for each mediator: (1) mistrust/abuse schemas, (2) abandonment schemas, and (3) defectiveness/shame schemas. Parental warmth and control were entered in the first step of each analysis in which PA was an independent variable.

Mistrust/abuse. The first step to test for mediation, that the IV predicts the DV, was established in the previous analysis. PA predicted mistrust/abuse schema, ANOVA $F(5,304) = 10.48$, $p < .001$, $R^2 = .15$. When considered with the parenting variables, PA was the only significant predictor ($\beta = .30$). MA schemas predicted interpersonal conflict ($\beta = .49$), ANOVA $F(1,362) = 116.35$, $p < .001$, $R^2 = .24$. In the final step, only paternal warmth ($\beta = -.15$, $p = .01$) and MA schemas ($\beta = .42$, $p < .001$) were significant predictors of interpersonal conflict, and the impact of PA was not statistically significant ($\beta = .15$, $p = .06$), ANOVA $F(6,302) = 23.72$, $p < .001$, $R^2 = .32$, suggesting that MA schemas mediated the relation between PA and adult interpersonal conflict (see Figure 1).

Abandonment. PA predicted abandonment, ANOVA $F(5,302) = 13.35$, $p < .001$, $R^2 = .18$. When considered with the parenting variables, PA was the only significant predictor ($\beta = .48$). Abandonment predicted conflict ($\beta = .39$), ANOVA $F(1,360) = 62.72$, $p < .001$, $R^2 = .15$. In the final step, only paternal warmth ($\beta = -.17$, $p = .01$) and AB schemas ($\beta = .31$, $p < .001$) were significant predictors of interpersonal conflict, and

FIGURE 1. Early maladaptive schemas fully mediate and partially mediate the relationship between childhood psychological abuse and adult interpersonal conflict

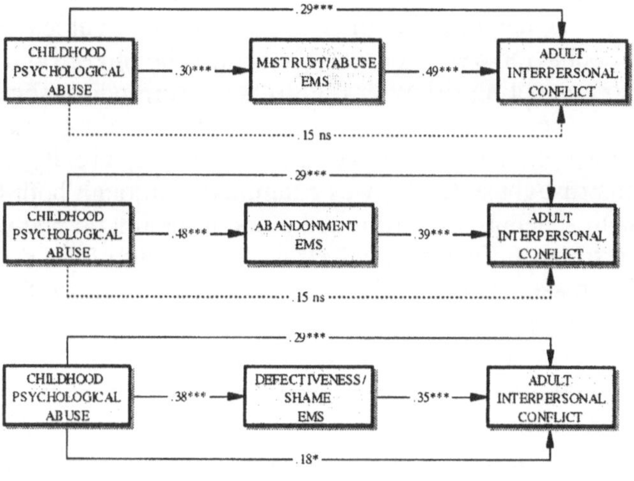

Note. The top line between psychological abuse and interpersonal conflict displays the standardized coefficient without the mediator present. The bottom line between psychological abuse and interpersonal conflict displays the standardized coefficient with each mediator present.
*** Indicates significance at the $p < .001$ level. * Indicates significance at the $p < .05$ level.

the impact of PA was not statistically significant (β = .15, p = .10), ANOVA $F(6,300)$ = 16.09, p < .001, R^2 = .24, suggesting that AB schemas mediated the relation between PA and adult interpersonal conflict (see Figure 1).

Defectiveness/shame. PA predicted defectiveness/shame schemas, ANOVA $F(5,302)$ = 7.06, p < .001, R^2 = .11. When considered with the parenting variables, PA was the only significant predictor (β = .38). DS schemas predicted conflict (β = .35), ANOVA $F(1,360)$ = 48.63, p < .001, R^2 = .12. In the final step, paternal warmth (β = –.14, p = .02), DS schemas (β = .31, p < .001), and PA (β = .18, p = .04) were all significant predictors of interpersonal conflict, ANOVA $F(6,300)$ = 17.21, p < .001, R^2 = .24. Results of a Sobel's test (Preacher & Leonardelli, 2001), t = 3.35, p < .001, indicated a significant reduction in impact of PA on interpersonal conflict (β = .29 in absence of mediator, β = .18 in presence of mediator), suggesting that DS schemas partially mediated the relation between PA and adult interpersonal conflict (see Figure 1).

Tests of Mediation: Interpersonal Behavior

The second set of analyses aimed to test whether coping style, in the form of interpersonal behavior, mediated the relation between early maladaptive schemas and adult interpersonal conflict. Three types of interpersonal behavior were examined to reflect the three coping styles: overly accommodating behavior (i.e., schema surrender), social isolation behavior (i.e., schema avoidance), and domineering and controlling behavior (i.e., schema overcompensation). For brevity, only one schema, mistrust/abuse (MA), was examined. Although both MA and abandonment schemas were full mediators of the relation between PA and interpersonal conflict, MA beliefs were the focus of this set of analyses because these schemas had the strongest relationship with interpersonal conflict when all four EMS were considered (see Table 2).

Overly accommodating behavior. Mistrust/abuse schemas predicted interpersonal conflict, ANOVA $F(1,362)$ = 116.35, p < .001, R^2 = .24, MA β = .48., and overly accommodating behavior (OA), ANOVA $F(1,343)$ = 53.19, p < .001, R^2 = .13. OA predicted conflict (β = .30), ANOVA $F(1,340)$ = 32.71, p < .001, R^2 = .09. In the final step, MA schemas (β = .43, p < .001) and OA behavior (β = .14, p < .01) were significant predictors of interpersonal conflict, ANOVA $F(2,334)$ = 55.35, p < .001, R^2 = .25. Results of a Sobel's test, t = 2.55, p < .001, indicated a significant reduction in impact of PA on interpersonal conflict ($\beta = .48$ in absence of mediator, $\beta = .43$ in presence of mediator), suggesting that OA behavior partially mediated the relation between MA schemas and interpersonal conflict.

Social isolation. The first step to test for mediation was established in the previous analysis. MA schemas predicted social isolation (SI), ANOVA $F(1,344) = 88.37, p < .001, R^2 = .20$, and SI predicted ($\beta = .30$) conflict, ANOVA $F(1,340) = 32.71, p < .001, R^2 = .09$. In the final step, MA schemas ($\beta = .39, p < .001$) and SI ($\beta = .21, p < .01$) were significant predictors of interpersonal conflict, ANOVA $F(2,335) = 61.70, p < .001$, $R^2 = .27$. Results of a Sobel's test, $t = 3.71, p < .001$, indicated a significant reduction in impact of MA schemas on interpersonal conflict ($\beta = .48$ in absence of mediator, $\beta = .39$ in presence of mediator), suggesting that SI partially mediated the relation between MA schemas and interpersonal conflict.

Domineering and controlling behavior. MA schemas predicted ($\beta = .25$) domineering and controlling (DC) behavior, ANOVA $F(1,346) = 23.87, p < .001, R^2 = .07$, and DC ($\beta = .47$) predicted conflict, ANOVA $F(1,344) = 95.52, p < .001, R^2 = .22$. In the final step, MA schemas ($\beta = .39, p < .001$) and DC ($\beta = .37, p < .01$) were significant predictors of interpersonal conflict, ANOVA $F(2,338) = 94.07, p < .001$, $R^2 = .36$. Results of a Sobel's test, $t = 4.19, p < .001$, indicated a significant reduction in impact of MA schemas on interpersonal conflict ($\beta = .48$ in absence of mediator, $\beta = .39$ in presence of mediator), suggesting that DC behavior partially mediated the relation between MA schemas and interpersonal conflict.

DISCUSSION

The present study supports earlier findings suggesting that PA during childhood has a significant impact on adult interpersonal functioning. One previous study (Varia & Abidin, 1999) found that PA was associated with lower levels of spousal support and increased spousal conflict, but the present findings suggest an even broader pattern of interpersonal conflict. In the present study, higher levels of conflict were associated with higher levels of PA, as well as lower levels of parental warmth and higher levels of parental control. Findings suggest that conflict occurred across several contexts, including romantic relationships, friendships, and work or school-related relationships. Although less is known about the specific nature of the interpersonal conflict, it appears that those endorsing conflict may be involved in relationships that Briere (1998) characterized as "chaotic and emotionally upsetting" (p. 10).

It is important to identify and document the relation between childhood PA and later interpersonal problems; however, it is also critical to understand how abuse experiences may increase the likelihood of later problems. Young's theory of early maladaptive schemas (EMS) appears to be a viable framework, which may be used to understand deleterious consequences of negative childhood experiences, including PA. In the present study, PA was significantly associated with several EMS within the disconnection and rejection domain, including abandonment concerns, emotional deprivation, mistrust/abuse and defectiveness/shame. These associations support claims by Bernstein (2002) and are generally consistent with Cecero et al. (2004), who found that PA predicted mistrust/abuse and defectiveness/shame schemas. The present study suggests that individuals who experience PA during childhood have a tendency to develop beliefs that others around them are not trustworthy, that others will not provide adequate emotional support when called upon, and at worst, that others may abandon or even abuse them. Furthermore, there is some evidence that the impact of PA on beliefs extends beyond perceptions of others and includes beliefs that the self is flawed, defective, or shameful. Such beliefs, although maladaptive and often self-perpetuating, are also understandable reactions to childhood experiences of PA.

In the current study, EMS played a critical role in the long-term impact of PA. It appears that PA affects EMS, which in turn, impact interpersonal conflict. When considered together, only three of the four EMS (i.e., mistrust/abuse, abandonment, and defectiveness/shame) predicted interpersonal conflict. Furthermore, mistrust/abuse appeared to have the strongest association with conflict. However, all three of the EMS examined mediated or partially mediated the relation between childhood PA and interpersonal conflict in adulthood. This suggests that the long-term impact of PA is perpetuated through the individual's perception of the abusive experience, particularly in relation to expectations regarding love and trust in interpersonal relationships (Steele, 1986).

Young et al. (2003) also argue that behavior is influenced by the joint impact of EMS and coping style. To test this assumption, interpersonal behavior was examined as a mediator of EMS and interpersonal conflict. The relation between mistrust/abuse schemas and interpersonal conflict was mediated or partially mediated by three different patterns of interpersonal behavior: overly accommodating behavior (schema surrender), social isolation (schema avoidance), and domineering and controlling behavior (schema overcompensation). Domineering and controlling behavior explained an additional 12% of the variance in conflict after considering mistrust/abuse schemas, whereas overly accommodating behavior and social isolation did not explain a significant amount of variance (R^2 increased .01 for OA, .03 for SI). This suggests that domineering and controlling behavior may be a more important factor in interpersonal conflict experienced by those with a history of PA. Although statistically significant, overly accommodating behavior and social isolation may not be as relevant. Both submissive and avoidant behavior may be related to mistrust/abuse schemas, but these two patterns of behavior may be less likely than controlling behavior to contribute to interpersonal conflict.

Given that psychologically abusive behavior may lie on a continuum with acceptable parenting practices, it is important to examine the impact of parenting behavior when studying the long-term effects of PA. In the current study, parenting behaviors were highly correlated with PA. Moreover, paternal warmth continued to have a significant direct impact on interpersonal conflict even when PA and schemas were included in the model. Interestingly, maternal warmth did not have a significant impact on interpersonal conflict, contrary to the findings of at least one other study (Varia & Abidin, 1999). Past research has primarily focused on maternal variables when examining parenting behavior, with very few studies focusing on the impact of paternal behavior. Among the few studies conducted, paternal parenting behavior was a strong predictor of later mental health functioning for women (Hall, Peden, Rayens, & Beebe, 2004; Turner, Rose, & Cooper, 2005). Not only are negative aspects of parenting (low warmth, high control) risk factors for later psychological difficulties, these parenting styles overlap to some extent with psychological abuse. However, our findings also suggest that the outcomes of PA as assessed by the CAMI (DiLillo, 2003) differ from those associated with relatively "normal" parenting practices, providing evidence of divergent validity for this new instrument. Parenting behavior did not predict EMS when considered with PA, suggesting that PA is more salient to the development of EMS than general parenting style. Regardless, findings suggest that paternal warmth is an important factor in later adult functioning.

One limitation of the current study is the use of retrospective self-report measures to assess child abuse experiences and perceived parenting behavior, which may influence the accuracy of these reports. However, all questionnaires were comprised of behaviorally specific questions and completed anonymously in order to encourage optimal accuracy in respondents' reporting. Also, research suggests that one's subjective perception of abusive experiences, especially PA, is a particularly important predictor of later functioning (McGee et al., 1997). As predicted, the constructs studied here were all significantly correlated; however, this brings into question the distinctness of some constructs. Future studies should continue to examine distinctions between different EMS that are often associated with child maltreatment (e.g., abandonment, mistrust/abuse schemas) as well as to further examine the overlap between psychological abuse and general parenting style.

A further limitation of the current study is the homogeneity of the sample of college women, which may impact generalization of findings to other more diverse populations. Future research should replicate these findings in clinical and other more diverse community samples. The current study focused only on PA to the exclusion of other forms of abuse and neglect. While measuring and comparing all types of child maltreatment is outside the scope of this study, it would be beneficial to understand how other types of maltreatment impact and are associated with EMS and adult interpersonal conflict.

The current study focused on PA as a broad construct. In order to gain a more thorough understanding of the impact of PA, future research should examine specific aspects of PA (e.g., spurning/terrorizing) on adult interpersonal functioning. This knowledge may allow for a greater understanding of the impact of PA and for greater specificity when designing clinical interventions. Additionally, future research should examine the impact of multiple forms of abuse (e.g., sexual abuse, physical abuse, etc.) and neglect because types of child maltreatment frequently overlap (Higgins & McCabe, 2001). However, there has been evidence suggesting that the effect of PA is significant and may have a stronger impact on mistrust/abuse schemas than other forms of abuse (Cecero et al., 2004). Future studies should continue to examine the impact of various forms of abuse on schema development and adult interpersonal functioning.

REFERENCES

Baron, R. M., & Kenny, D. A. (1986). The moderator-mediator variable distinction in social psychological research: Conceptual, strategic, and statistical considerations. *Journal of Personality and Social Psychology, 51*(6), 1173-1182.

Bernstein, D. P. (2002). Cognitive therapy of personality disorders in patients with histories of emotional abuse or neglect. *Psychiatric Annals, 32*(10), 618-628.

Briere, J. (1998). *Inventory of altered self-capacities*. Odessa, FL: Psychological Assessment Resources.

Briere, J., & Runtz, M. (1988). Multivariate correlates of childhood psychological and physical maltreatment among university women. *Child Abuse and Neglect, 12*, 331-341.

Briere, J., & Runtz, M. (1990). Differential adult symptomatology associated with three types of child abuse histories. *Child Abuse and Neglect, 14*(3), 357-364.

Cecero, J. J., Nelson, J. D., & Gillie, J. M. (2004). Tools and tenets of schema therapy: Toward the construct validity of the early maladaptive schema questionnaire-research version (EMSQ-R). *Clinical Psychology and Psychotherapy, 11*, 344-357.

Cerezo, M. A., & Frias, D. (1994). Emotional and cognitive adjustment in abused children. *Child Abuse and Neglect, 18*(11), 923-932.

Claussen, A. I., & Crittenden, P. (1991). Physical and psychological maltreatment: Relations among types of maltreatment. *Child Abuse and Neglect, 15*, 5-18.

Clemmons, J. (2005). *Multiple forms of child maltreatment and abuse-specific characteristics: Relationships to adult adjustment*. Unpublished doctoral dissertation. University of Nebraska-Lincoln.

DiLillo, D. (2003). *The Computer Assisted Maltreatment Inventory (CAMI)*. Unpublished measure.

Gross, A. B., & Keller, H. R. (1992). Long-term consequences of childhood physical and psychological maltreatment. *Aggressive Behavior, 18*, 171-185.

Hall, L. A., Peden, A. R., Rayens, M. K., & Beebe, L. H. (2004). Parental bonding: A key factor for mental health of college women. *Issues in Mental Health Nursing, 25*, 277-291.

Hart, S. N., Brassard, M. R., Bineggeli, N. J., & Davidson, H. A. (2002). Psychological maltreatment. In J. E. B. Myers, L. Berliner, J. Briere, C. T. Hendrix, C. Jenny, & T. A. Reid (Eds.), *The APSAC handbook on child maltreatment* (2nd ed.). Thousand Oaks, CA: Sage Publications, Inc.

Higgins, D. J., & McCabe, M. P. (2001). Multiple forms of child abuse and neglect: Adult retrospective reports. *Aggression and Violent Behavior, 6*, 547-578.

Horowitz, L., Alden, L. E., Wiggins, J. S., & Pincus, A. L. (2000). *Inventory of Interpersonal Problems*. Psychological Corporation: Harcourt Assessment Company.

Kaufman, J. (1991). Depressive disorders in maltreated children. *Journal of the American Academy of Child and Adolescent Psychiatry, 30*(2), 257-265.

Krause, E. D., Mendelson, T., & Lynch, T. R. (2003). Childhood emotional invalidation and adult psychological distress: The mediating role of emotional inhibition. *Child Abuse and Neglect, 27*, 199-213.

McGee, R. A., Wolfe, D.A., & Wilson, S. K. (1997). Multiple childhood maltreatment experiences and adolescent behavior problems: Adolescents' perspectives. *Development and Psychopathology, 9*, 131-149.

Moran, P. M., Bifulco, A., Ball, C., Jacobs, C., & Benaim, K. (2002). Exploring psychological abuse in childhood: I. Developing a new interview scale. *Bulletin of the Menninger Clinic, 66*, 213-240.

Mullen, P. E., Martin, J. L., Anderson, J. C., Romans, S. E., & Herbison, G. P. (1996). The long-term impact of the physical, emotional, and sexual abuse of children: A community study. *Child Abuse and Neglect, 20*(1), 7-21.

Nash, C. L., DiLillo, D., Messman-Moore, T., & Rinkol, S. (2002, November). *The Computer Assisted Maltreatment Inventory (CAMI): An Investigation of test-retest reliability and criterion validity*. Paper presented at the 36th annual meeting of the Association for the Advancement of Behavior Therapy, Reno, Nevada.

Nash, C. L. (2005). *Reliability, validity, and factor structure of the psychological abuse and neglect scales of the Computer Assisted Maltreatment Inventory*. Unpublished doctoral dissertation. University of Nebraska-Lincoln.

Parker, G., Tupling, H., & Brown, L. B. (1979). A parental bonding instrument. *British Journal of Medical Psychology, 52*, 1-10.

Preacher, K. J., & Leonardelli, G. J. (2001, March). Calculation for the Sobel test: An interactive calculation tool for mediation tests [Computer software]. Available from http://www.quantpsy.org.

Scher, C. D., Forde, D. R., McQuaid, J. R., & Stein, M. B. (2004). Prevalence and demographic correlates of childhood maltreatment in an adult community sample. *Child Abuse and Neglect, 28*, 167-180.

Schmidt, N. B., Joiner, T. E., Young, J. E., & Telch, M. J. (1995). The schema questionnaire: Investigation of psychometric properties and the hierarchical structure of a measure of maladaptive schemas. *Cognitive Therapy and Research, 19*(3), 295-321.

Spertus, I. L., Yehuda, R., Wong, C. M., Halligan, S., & Seremetis, S. V. (2003). Childhood emotional abuse and neglect as predictors of psychological and physical symptoms in women presenting to a primary care practice. *Child Abuse and Neglect, 27*, 1247-1258.

Steele, B. F. (1986). Notes on the lasting effect of early child abuse throughout the life cycle. *Child Abuse and Neglect, 10*, 228-291.

Straus, M. A., & Field, C. J. (2003). Psychological aggression by American parents: Data on prevalence, chronicity and severity. *Journal of Marriage and Family, 65*, 795-808.

Turner, H. M., Rose, K. S., & Cooper, M. L. (2005). Schema and parental bonding in overweight and nonoverweight female adolescents. *International Journal of Obesity, 29*(4), 381-387.

Varia, R., & Abidin, R. R. (1999). The minimizing style: Perceptions of psychological abuse and quality of past and current relationships. *Child Abuse and Neglect, 23*(11), 1041-1055.

Vissing, Y. M., Straus, M. A., Gelles, R. J., & Harrop, J. W. (1991). Verbal aggression by parents and psychosocial problems of children. *Child Abuse and Neglect, 15*, 223-238.

Young, J. E., Klosko, J. S., & Weishaar, J. E. (2003). *Schema therapy: A practitioner's guide*. New York: Guilford Press.

doi:10.1300/J135v07n02_05

The Impact of Childhood Psychological Maltreatment on Interpersonal Schemas and Subsequent Experiences of Relationship Aggression

Emily Crawford
Margaret O'Dougherty Wright

SUMMARY. The relationships between child psychological maltreatment, interpersonal schemas, and adult relationship aggression were explored in 301 college men and women. Participants completed questionnaires assessing a history of child abuse, current maladaptive schemas, adult intimate partner victimization, and perpetration of adult aggression. Child psychological maltreatment predicted both perpetration and revictimization experiences of adult interpersonal aggression even after controlling for other childhood abuse experiences. The schemas of mistrust, self-sacrifice, and emotional inhibition fully mediated the relationship between child psychological maltreatment and adult intimate partner victimization. The schemas of mistrust, entitlement, emotional

---

Address correspondence to: Emily Crawford, Department of Psychology, Psychology Building, Room 100 G, Miami University, Oxford, OH 45056 (E-mail: crawfoeb@muohio.edu).

The authors would like to thank Zachary Birchmeier, PhD, for his assistance with the statistical analysis.

[Haworth co-indexing entry note]: "The Impact of Childhood Psychological Maltreatment on Interpersonal Schemas and Subsequent Experiences of Relationship Aggression." Crawford, Emily, and Margaret O'Dougherty Wright. Co-published simultaneously in *Journal of Emotional Abuse* (The Haworth Maltreatment & Trauma Press, an imprint of The Haworth Press, Inc.) Vol. 7, No. 2, 2007, pp. 93-116; and: *Childhood Emotional Abuse: Mediating and Moderating Processes Affecting Long-Term Impact* (ed: Margaret O'Dougherty Wright) The Haworth Maltreatment & Trauma Press, an imprint of The Haworth Press, Inc., 2007, pp. 93-116. Single or multiple copies of this article are available for a fee from The Haworth Document Delivery Service [1-800-HAWORTH, 9:00 a.m. - 5:00 p.m. (EST). E-mail address: docdelivery@haworthpress.com].

Available online at http://jea.haworthpress.com

doi:10.1300/J135v07n02_06

inhibition, and insufficient self-control partially mediated the relationship between child psychological maltreatment and one's own perpetration of aggression. Implications for intervening with young adults at risk for relationship aggression are discussed. doi:10.1300/J135v07n02_06

KEYWORDS. Child psychological maltreatment, interpersonal schemas, adult intimate partner violence, revictimization

> Children make meaning of their abuse in many ways . . . when we think of maltreatment outcomes as responses to how children explain what has happened to them, distinctions between abuse categories become somewhat artificial . . . although we may treat the physical manifestations of abuse, it is the psychological manifestations that will continue to haunt us . . . in our mental hospitals, in violence in our streets, and in our families. (Newberger 1991, as quoted in Sanders & Becker-Lausen, 1995, p. 320)

INTRODUCTION

Psychological maltreatment refers to a pattern of emotional abuse or neglect, examples of which include hostile rejecting of the child, degrading (e.g., defining the child as a failure), terrorizing, corrupting, denying emotional responsiveness, isolating the child, or failing to provide for the child's needs (APSAC, 1995, as cited in Glaser, 2002). Psychological maltreatment is the most commonly occurring form of child abuse. This is because while psychological maltreatment does occur in isolation (these cases of abuse are seldom reported), many cases of physical and sexual abuse also have an element of emotional abuse, and the impact from this type of abuse may persist long after the physical injuries have healed (Davis, Petretic-Jackson, & Ting, 2001; Hamarman & Bernet, 2000; Higgins & McCabe, 2001; Manly, Kim, Rogosch, & Cicchetti, 2001; Schneider, Ross, Graham, & Zielinski, 2005).

Psychological maltreatment has been identified as a significant predictor of many long-term intrapsychic consequences such as low self-esteem, self-depreciation, suicidal ideation, personality disorders, and eating psychopathology (Bierer et al., 2003; Bifulco, Moran, Baines, Bunn, & Stanford, 2002; Higgins & McCabe, 2000; Kent & Waller, 2000; McGee, Wolfe, & Wilson, 1997). Psychological maltreatment may be the form of abuse that is most predictive of a cognitive vulnerability to depression. This refers to the tendency to make internal, stable, and global negative attributions about the self and to infer negative consequences for the self following an unpleasant life event (Gibb et al., 2001). It is not surprising that this vulnerability is likely to develop among survivors of psychological maltreatment since their perpetrators often directly supply them with damaging cognitions about themselves. The emotional invalidation that victims of child psychological maltreatment often endure is also strongly associated with symptoms of depression and anxiety and can result in significant emotional inhibition (Krause, Mendelson, & Lynch, 2003). The present study seeks to expand our understanding of how inhibiting one's emotions and internalizing negative feelings and beliefs about the self may affect interpersonal relationships.

ADULT RELATIONSHIP AGGRESSION

Although there has been little direct research attention given to the impact of such treatment on subsequent interpersonal relationships, psychological abuse occurs in an interpersonal context and thus may increase the risk of later difficulty with trust and intimacy. The inhibition of emotional expression that can follow psychologically abusive treatment may contribute to difficulties in intimate relationships in which the ability to identify and respectfully assert one's needs and to negotiate conflict is essential to the maintenance of a mutually healthy and satisfying connection. A recent study of adults with a history of childhood verbal abuse revealed that they were more likely than other adults to express a wish for distance from others (Drapeau & Perry, 2004). It may be that some individuals who experience child psychological maltreatment come to believe that they do not have the ability to avoid conflict with others. Such a belief may, in some cases, lead to withdrawal from intimate relationships.

Although research on the specific long-term interpersonal consequences of psychological abuse is sparse, data that does exist suggests that couple relationships may be one of the most challenging interpersonal interactions for child abuse survivors. There is some evidence to suggest that individuals with a history of boundary violations (e.g., the experience of parental role reversal) are more likely to act in their intimate relationships as the aggressor, the victim, or both (Linder & Collins, 2005). In addition, we know that experiencing other forms of child abuse is related to subsequent experiences of adult intimate partner violence (Lang, Stein, Kennedy, & Foy, 2004; Whitfield, Anda, Dube, & Felitti, 2003) and a heightened probability of sexual revictimization (Arata, 2002; Messman-Moore & Long, 2003). Women who reported having experienced physical abuse as children, as well as women who indicated that they witnessed domestic violence, appeared to be at increased risk for being physically and emotionally abused by a partner in adulthood (Bensley, Van Eenwyk, & Simmons, 2003). Also, compared to women without a sexual abuse history, child sexual abuse survivors were more likely to report that their adult intimate relationships had involved incidents of both initiating and receiving physical aggression. In other words, a sexual abuse history was related to increased risk for mutually inflicted couple violence (DiLillo, Giuffre, Tremblay, & Peterson, 2001). Thus, there is evidence that children who experience physical and/or sexual abuse are at risk for becoming involved in intimate adult relationships that are characterized by abuse. The present study seeks to explore the unique impact that experiences of child psychological maltreatment may have on intimate relationships in adulthood.

Interpersonal Schemas

Attachment theory, through its characterization of internal representational models, offers a valuable organizing framework for understanding later patterns of maladaptive interpersonal relationships. A central concept of attachment theory is that children form representational models of attachment figures, of themselves, and of themselves in relation to others based on their relationship history with their primary caregivers (Bowlby, 1982). These working models, called schemas, form templates for how the person expects to be treated by others based on how he or she was treated and what he or she brings to relationships. Representational models are typically constructed in terms of beliefs regarding the degree to which the "self" is thought to be acceptable and worthy of love and the "other" is believed to be responsive and able to be depended upon to provide love and care. These relational schemas guide the interpretation of relationship information and influence relationship behavior (Baldwin, 1992).

Exposure to experiences of emotional abuse in childhood is likely to threaten the security of these attachment relationships and may result in maladaptive models of self and self-in-relation to others (Cicchetti & Toth, 2000; Collins, Guichard, Ford, & Feeney, 2004). In addition to the intrapsychic effects of psychological maltreatment discussed earlier, when individuals have experienced negative and abusive early relationships, abuse-related attachment schemas may become activated later in life in intimate relationships. Such individuals are thus at risk for continued abuse from a partner, or alternatively, individuals who hold such schemas may be at risk for becoming abusive (Cicchetti & Toth, 1995; 2000).

However, not every child abuse survivor will inevitably experience victimization in his or her adult relationships. Cloitre, Cohen, and Scarvalone (2002) provide us with evidence of the interpersonal schemas that survivors of abuse hold in adulthood as a compelling explanation for the important differences among survivors with regard to the likelihood of experiencing subsequent victimization. Specifically, female child sexual abuse survivors who expected others to respond in a hostile and controlling manner regardless of their own actions were more likely than other survivors to experience sexual revictimization as an adult. In contrast, child sexual abuse survivors who were not revictimized in adulthood were able to refrain from generalizing their negative parental schemas of others as untrustworthy and hostile to their current romantic partners. Unfortunately, very little is known about how such individuals learned to form new relational schemas.

Facilitating exploration of such schemas, Young, Klosko, and Weishaar (2003) have recently developed a questionnaire that specifically assesses early maladaptive schemas (EMSs), which they characterize as pervasive organizing principles by which people make sense of early life experiences that were typically abusive or neglectful. Young and colleagues further postulate that child abuse survivors may cope with EMSs in different ways, such as by surrender, avoidance, or overcompensation. The child abuse survivor who surrenders to a mistrust/abuse schema may find the role of victim in an intimate relationship familiar, choose a partner that represents an abusive parent, and not recognize that there are alternative, healthier ways of being in relationship with others. The survivor who avoids confronting the constant expectation that others are going to hurt him or her may withdraw from others and will likely present with loneliness and depressive symptoms. Finally, the survivor who overcompensates for a mistrust/abuse schema may lash out in anger at the slightest provocation that signals that abuse is apt to take place. Such a coping strategy may result in the survivor being verbally or physically abusive to significant others. This coping strategy is likely to alienate others and may even result in retaliation, which would then confirm the survivor's original expectations. In this way, EMSs can be self-perpetuating.

Goals of the Present Study

Prior research has indicated that certain EMSs partially mediate the relationship between undergraduate students' retrospective perceptions of parenting as being uncaring or overprotective and current depressive symptoms (Harris & Curtin, 2002). We seek to expand on this research in the current study by focusing on the impact of child psychological abuse on the development of EMSs and exploring the relationships between psychological maltreatment, EMSs, and later adult interpersonal relationships. Specific questions addressed were: How do adult survivors of childhood psychological maltreatment experience themselves in relation to others? What kinds of interpersonal difficulties are predicted from the interpersonal schemas they hold? In particular, is the experience of abusive behaviors in intimate adult relationships (either as a victim or a perpetrator of abuse) related to child psychological maltreatment, and if so, do EMSs provide a plausible explanation for this relationship?

It was hypothesized that after controlling for the experiences of physical abuse, sexual abuse, and problematic parental alcohol use, experiences of psychological maltreatment would still predict self-reported experiences as a victim of adult intimate partner abuse, in addition to self-reported experiences as a perpetrator of interpersonal aggression. It was also hypothesized that psychological maltreatment would predict the development of specific EMSs, which might mediate the relationship between psychological maltreatment and adult intimate partner victimization experiences as well as the relationship between psychological maltreatment and one's own perpetration of aggression.

METHOD

Participants

Participants were male and female students enrolled in Introductory Psychology at an undergraduate university in the Midwest. Students signed up for this study through an on-line program and received two credits toward their course requirements of 12 research credits as compensation. A total of 351 students participated in the study. Of these participants, 50 were dropped from the analyses due to incomplete data, leaving a sample of 301 (143 men and 158 women). The mean age of the participants was 20.37 years, with 52.5% of the sample indicating that they were female. The percentages of participants by ethnicity are reported as follows: 284 (94.4%) Caucasian, 8 (2.7%) African-American, 2 (.7%) Native-American, 2 (.7%) Asian-American, 7 (2.3%) Hispanic, and 4 (1.3%) "other race." The mean reported annual income for the participants' parents was between $50,000 and $75,000.

Measures and Procedure

This study received the approval of the University's institutional review board. Following both a written and verbal informed consent, each participant completed a questionnaire containing, in order, demographic measures, the Index of Dating Abuse (Walter & McIntosh, 1981), the Children of Alcoholics Screening Test-6 (CAST-6; Hodgins, Maticka-Tyndale, El-Guebaly, & West, 1993), the Lifetime Experiences Questionnaire (Gibb et al., 2001), Young's Schema Questionnaire (Young, 1999), and the Aggression Questionnaire (Buss & Perry, 1992). Each of these measures is described in more detail in the following paragraphs.

Index of Dating Abuse. The Index of Dating Abuse (IDA) is a 31-item questionnaire adapted from the Index of Spousal Abuse (Walter & McIntosh, 1981) by removing the item "My partner is stingy in giving me enough money to run our house" and rewording the questions to make the items appropriate for both males and females to respond. This measure contains items designed to assess physical, emotional, and sexual abuse between adult intimate partners (e.g., "My partner slaps me around my face and head," "My partner screams and yells at me," and "My partner demands sex whether I want it or not"). Participants were asked to indicate the degree to which each event may have occurred in any of their intimate relationships since age 18 on a scale of 1-5 with 1 meaning "never" and 5 meaning "very frequently." Ratings were averaged to form a total score on this measure. Cronbach's alpha for the measure in this sample is .96.

Children of Alcoholics Screening Test (CAST-6). This 6-item true/false measure is designed to assess whether or not participants perceived alcohol abuse or dependence in their parents. This short form of the CAST has been shown to discriminate between adult children of alcoholics and adult children of non-alcoholics as well as does the full 30 item measure. Participants' ratings were summed to form a total score on this measure. Cronbach's alpha was .86 for student samples as reported by Hodgins and colleagues (1993).

Lifetime Experiences Questionnaire. The Lifetime Experiences Questionnaire (LEQ) is an 82-item measure containing items that inquire about various forms of childhood emotional abuse and neglect, physical abuse and neglect, and sexual abuse experiences that occurred prior to age 15. For example, participants responded to questions such as, "Did anyone humiliate or demean you in the presence of other people?" "Were you ever beaten up?" and "Did any adult or someone more than five years older than you ever touch you in a sexual way?" Participants were then asked to report how often each situation occurred prior to age 15, from "never" to "more than 20 times." Continuous variables for each type of child abuse (emotional abuse/neglect, physical abuse/neglect, and sexual abuse) were created by averaging the participants' frequency ratings across the items designed to measure each type of abuse. Alpha ratings in this sample were .86 for emotional abuse/neglect, .70 for physical abuse/neglect, and .80 for sexual abuse, which are similar to the ratings found in the research by Gibb and colleagues (2001).

Young's Schema Questionnaire. Young's Schema Questionnaire (YSQ) is a 205-item measure developed to assess the degree to which participants adhere to the 16 early maladaptive schemas described by Young (1999). These schemas are named: emotional deprivation, abandonment, mistrust/abuse, social isolation, defectiveness/shame, social undesirability, failure to achieve, functional dependence/independence, vulnerability to harm and illness, enmeshment, subjugation, self-sacrifice, emotional inhibition, unrelenting standards, entitlement, and insufficient self-control/self-discipline. Examples of items are: "I feel that people will take advantage of me" (mistrust/abuse), "I'm the one who usually ends of taking care of the people I'm close to" (self-sacrifice), "I'm special and shouldn't have to accept many of the restrictions placed on other people" (entitlement), "I find it embarrassing to express my feelings to others" (emotional inhibition), and "I often do things impulsively that I later regret" (insufficient self-control/self-discipline). Participants were asked to rate each item on a scale of 1 ("completely untrue") to 6 ("completely true"). Continuous variables for each schema were created by averaging the participants' ratings across the items designed to assess each schema. Cronbach's alpha for the measure in this sample is .98.

Aggression Questionnaire. The Aggression Questionnaire (AQ) we used in this sample contains the 28 items developed by Buss and Perry (1992) in addition to several questions adapted from the Sexual Experiences Survey (Koss and Gidycz, 1982). Items inquired about participants' perpetration of acts of physical, verbal, and sexual aggression (e.g., "If somebody hits me, I hit back" and "I have threatened people I know"). Participants were asked to rate each item on a scale of 1 to 5, with 1 meaning "not at all characteristic" and 5 meaning "very characteristic." Ratings were averaged to form a total score on this measure. Cronbach's alpha for the measure in this sample is .93.

RESULTS

Psychological Maltreatment and Adult Relationships

Hierarchical regression analyses provided support for our hypotheses that emotional abuse/neglect would emerge as an independent predictor of both victimization and perpetration of interpersonal aggression in adulthood. In this analysis, gender and income were entered into the first step, followed by problematic parental alcohol use and child sexual abuse in the second step, child physical abuse and neglect in the third step, and child emotional abuse and neglect in the fourth step. This allowed examination of the additional predictive power of child emotional abuse experiences after controlling for the other demographic and family environment variables. The total model was significant in predicting victimization experiences by an adult intimate partner (as measured by the total score on the IDA), accounting for 12.5% of the variance, $F(6, 231) = 5.37, p < .0001$. Gender, child sexual abuse, and child emotional abuse and neglect emerged as significant predictors. Experiences of emotional abuse and neglect did contribute unique variance to the prediction of victimization by an adult intimate partner ($t = 3.20, p < .002$), accounting for 4% of the R^2 change (illustrated in Table 1). This model was also significant in predicting self-reported perpetration of aggression (as measured by the total score on the AQ), accounting for 17.7% of the variance, $F(6, 228) = 7.95$, $p < .0001$. Gender, income, child physical abuse and neglect, and child emotional abuse and neglect all emerged as significant predictors. Emotional abuse and neglect did contribute unique variance to the prediction of self-reported perpetration of aggression ($t = 2.36, p < .02$), accounting for 2.1% of the R^2 change (illustrated in Table 2).

TABLE 1. Hierarchical Regression Analyses Exploring the Impact of Child Maltreatment on Experiences of Adult Intimate Partner Victimization

Variables		R^2 change	β	*t*-scores
Step 1	gender		–.123	–1.94*
	income	.01	–.022	–.336
Step 2	parental alcoholism		.051	.803
	child sexual abuse	.07**	.232	3.38**
Step 3	child physical abuse and neglect	.00	–.173	–2.06*
Step 4	child emotional abuse and neglect	.04**	.263	3.20**

* $p < .05$
** $p < .01$

TABLE 2. Hierarchical Regression Analyses Exploring the Impact of Child Maltreatment on Experiences of Self-Reported Adult Perpetration of Aggression

Variables		R^2 change	β	*t*-scores
Step 1	gender		–.160	–2.57**
	income	.04**	.164	2.58**
Step 2	parental alcoholism		–.019	–.313
	child sexual abuse	.05**	.098	1.46**
Step 3	child physical abuse and neglect	.07**	.187	2.32*
Step 4	child emotional abuse and neglect	.02*	.189	2.36*

* $p < .05$
** $p < .01$

Interpersonal Schemas and Adult Relationships

Young's 16 schemas were examined as possible predictors of experiences of adult intimate partner victimization (as measured by the IDA). A forward regression analysis predicting the total score on the IDA was conducted. All schemas were entered in a single step, with the exception of three schemas (abandonment, defectiveness/shame, and failure to achieve) that correlated highly (above .70) with several other schemas and also had VIF scores above 4.0. These three schemas were dropped from all analyses in order to reduce the possibility of multicollinearity (Stevens, 2002). Subsequent pairwise correlations between the schemas were all less than .70. The model predicting experiences of adult intimate partner victimization was significant and accounted for 19.1% of the variance, $F(3, 267) = 20.84, p < .0001$. Higher scores on the schema of mistrust ($t = 2.51, p < .01$), the schema of self-sacrifice ($t = 2.57, p < .01$), and the schema of emotional inhibition ($t = 2.28, p < .02$) were all related to a greater number of reported experiences of adult intimate partner victimization.

Young's schemas were also examined in a forward regression analysis as potential predictors of self-reported perpetration of aggression (as measured by the AQ). The model was significant and accounted for 42.6% of the variance, $F(4, 265) = 48.42, p < .0001$. Higher scores on the schema of mistrust ($t = 2.98, p < .003$), the schema of entitlement ($t = 3.05, p < .003$), the schema of emotional inhibition ($t = 2.04, p < .04$), and the schema of insufficient self-control ($t = 4.03, p < .0001$) were all related to a greater number of reported perpetrations of aggression.

Psychological Maltreatment, Interpersonal Schemas, and Adult Relationships

A series of hierarchical multiple regression analyses were completed in order to test the possibility that the schemas of mistrust, self-sacrifice, and emotional inhibition might mediate the relationship between child psychological maltreatment and adult intimate partner victimization experiences. The relationships in this model are represented in Figure 1.

According to Baron and Kenny's (1986) model, evidence for mediation would exist if the following four criteria were met: First, child psychological maltreatment should significantly predict adult intimate partner victimization. This first criterion was met in our sample, such that psychological maltreatment accounted for 3.5% of the variance in adult intimate partner victimization, $F(1, 286) = 10.47, p <.001$. Second, child psychological maltreatment must predict each schema. Indeed, child psychological maltreatment accounted for 17.6% of the variance in the schema of mistrust, $F(1, 292) = 61.94, p < .0001$. Child psychological maltreatment accounted for 9.4% of the variance in the self-sacrifice schema, $F(1, 288) = 29.74, p < .0001$, and 10.6% of the variance in emotional inhibition, $F(1, 292) = 34.54, p < .0001$. The third criterion required for mediation is that the schemas must predict adult intimate partner victimization. This criterion was also fulfilled in our sample (see forward regression analyses reported under "Interpersonal Schemas and Adult Relationships"). Finally, for the schemas to emerge as mediators, the impact of psychological maltreatment on adult intimate partner victimization should be less when each of the schemas are included in the regressions. Indeed, psychological maltreatment was no longer a

FIGURE 1. Mediation analysis predicting experiences of intimate partner victimization from child psychological maltreatment and schemas of mistrust, self-sacrifice, and emotional inhibition

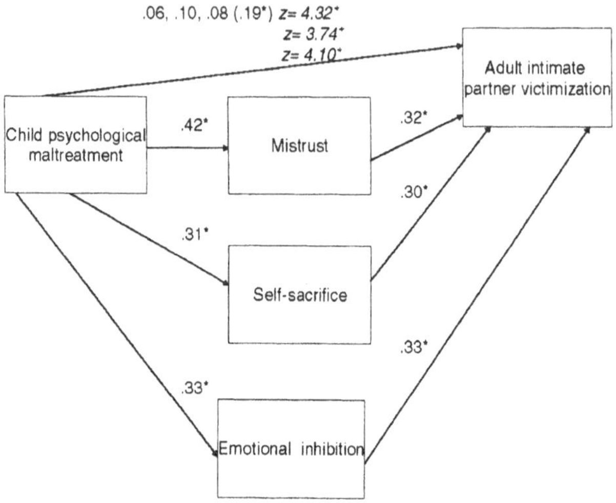

All estimates are standardized.
The estimate in the parenthesis is pre-mediation.
* $p < .01$

significant predictor of adult intimate partner victimization when each of the schemas was included in the regressions. In addition, the results of several Sobel tests indicated full mediation (see z scores in Figure 1).

Together, experiences of child psychological maltreatment and the schema of mistrust accounted for 11.9% of the variance in total IDA scores, $F(2, 283) = 18.92, p < .0001$. The complete model with child psychological maltreatment and the schema of self-sacrifice accounted for 11.9% of the variance in IDA, $F(2, 279) = 18.79$, $p < .0001$, and the model with child psychological maltreatment and the schema of emotional inhibition accounted for 13.3% of the variance in IDA, $F(2, 283) = 21.64, p < .0001$. Thus, evidence for full mediation emerged, such that it appeared that the association between experiences of child psychological maltreatment and experiences of adult intimate partner victimization was mediated by holding a schema of mistrust. Results also suggested that the relationship between psychological maltreatment and experiences of adult intimate partner victimization was mediated by both the schema of self-sacrifice and by the schema of emotional inhibition.

Hierarchical multiple regression analyses also provided some support for the hypothesis that the schemas that predicted self-reported perpetration of aggression in this sample (mistrust, entitlement, emotional inhibition, and insufficient self-control) mediated the relationship between child psychological maltreatment and one's own adulthood perpetration of aggression. The relationships in this model are represented in Figure 2. The first criterion in Baron and Kenny's (1986) mediation model was met in our sample, such that psychological maltreatment accounted for 9.8% of the variance in self-reported adult perpetration of aggression, $F(1, 280) = 30.38, p < .0001$. Second, child psychological maltreatment accounted for 3.3% of the variance in the entitlement schema, $F(1, 292) = 9.81, p < .002$, and 7.2% of the variance in insufficient self-control, $F(1, 290) = 22.47, p < .0001$. As previously reported (see above), psychological maltreatment also accounted for a significant amount of the

FIGURE 2. Mediation analysis predicting self-reported adult perpetration of interpersonal aggression from child psychological maltreatment and schemas of mistrust, entitlement, insufficient self-control, and emotional inhibition

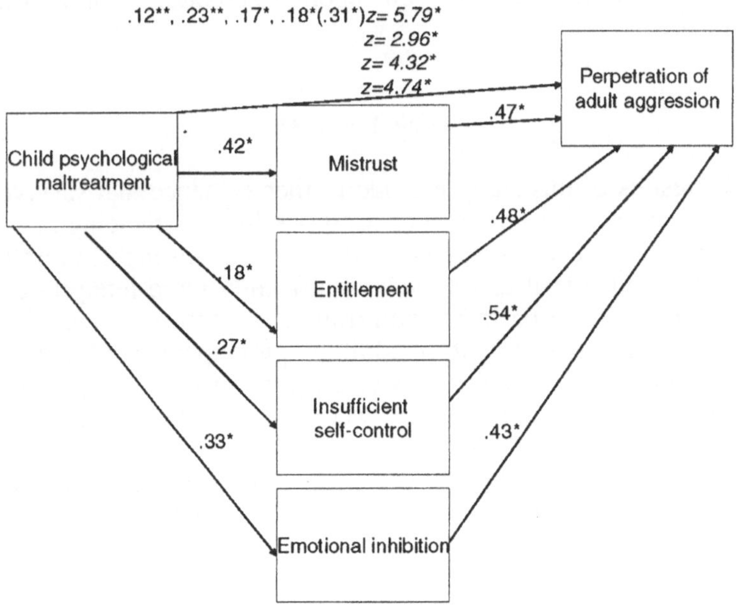

All estimates are standardized.
The estimate in the parenthesis is pre-mediation.
** $p < .05$
* $p < .01$

variance in mistrust (17.6%) and emotional inhibition (10.6%). The association of psychological maltreatment and self-reported adult perpetration of aggression was reduced when each of the schemas were included in the regressions. In addition, the results of several Sobel tests indicated partial mediation (see z scores in Figure 2).

Together, experiences of child psychological maltreatment and the schema of mistrust accounted for 28.5% of the variance in total AQ scores, $F(2, 278) = 54.99$, $p < .0001$. The complete model with child psychological maltreatment and the schema of entitlement accounted for 31.9% of the variance in AQ, $F(2, 277) = 64.54$, $p < .0001$, the model with child psychological maltreatment and the schema of emotional inhibition accounted for 26.7% of the variance in AQ, $F(2, 278) = 50.21$, $p < .0001$, and the model with child psychological maltreatment and the schema of insufficient self-control accounted for 36.6% of the variance in AQ, $F(2, 276) = 78.99$, $p < .0001$. Thus, evidence for partial mediation emerged, such that it appeared that the schemas of mistrust, entitlement, emotional inhibition, and insufficient self-control were all partial mediators of the association between experiences of child psychological maltreatment and self-reported perpetration of adult interpersonal aggression.

DISCUSSION

The results of this study provide further evidence that survivors of child abuse or neglect are at increased risk for experiencing adult intimate partner violence. Specifically, the young adults in this sample who survived child sexual abuse were significantly more likely to experience adult intimate partner victimization, as were survivors of child psychological maltreatment. In addition, participants who had experienced child physical abuse, as well as participants who had endured child psychological maltreatment, were significantly more likely to report that they had acted as the aggressor in their adult relationships. Surprisingly, survivors of child physical abuse were actually *less* likely to indicate experiences of adult intimate partner victimization, though this variable did not account for a significant amount of R^2 change in the regression model. It is also noteworthy that males reported significantly more experiences of both adult intimate partner victimization as well as adult perpetration of aggression compared to females. While reports of higher rates of male perpetration of aggression were expected based on prior research (Ehrensaft et al., 2003; Stith et al., 2000; Straus, Gelles, &

Steinmetz, 1980), the finding that men would also report more victimization experiences in dating was unexpected. However, other research reported in this special issue has also found that men report higher rates of interpersonal mistreatment compared to women (Newton & Weigel, 2007).

Consistent with our hypothesis that psychological abuse is harmful in its own right, child psychological maltreatment did account for a significant amount of the R^2 change in both adult intimate partner victimization experiences as well as self-reported acts of adult aggression even after controlling for gender, income, problematic parental alcohol use, and other forms of child abuse. In fact, child psychological maltreatment actually accounted for more of the R^2 change in adult intimate partner victimization than did child physical abuse. This finding is consistent with the suggestions of prior researchers that the psychological abuse inherent in all forms of child abuse may explain many of the long-term consequences of an abusive childhood (Fortin & Chamberland, 1995).

Of course, there is considerable variability in the association between child victimization experiences and adult relationship aggression. This study's findings support the mediational role that specific interpersonal schemas play in the development of relationship abuse. Individuals who had negative experiences with their parents and who internalized these early experiences in the form of maladaptive schemas were at heightened risk of experiencing similar negative interactions in their romantic partner relationships. Specifically, the schemas of mistrust, self-sacrifice, and emotional inhibition all emerged as full mediators of the relationship between psychological maltreatment and experiences of adult intimate partner victimization. In other words, survivors of child psychological maltreatment who believed that others would respond to them in an abusive manner (such survivors hold a schema of mistrust) were more likely to have these expectations realized by abusive adult intimate partners. Also, child psychological maltreatment survivors who consistently placed others' needs above their own may have learned that doing so appeased their abuser at times and thus served as a survival mechanism in childhood. However, while possibly effective in obtaining much needed approval, such a pattern of compulsive caregiving may be associated with deleterious long-term consequences (Bellow, Boris, Larrieu, Lewis, & Elliot, 2005). Unfortunately, as demonstrated in this study, psychological abuse survivors who continued to be self-sacrificing were more likely to experience victimization perpetrated by their adult intimate partners.

Our findings are also consistent with prior research demonstrating that the emotional invalidation that victims of child emotional abuse often experience strongly predicts adult adjustment difficulties. Emotional inhibition refers to both the avoidance of emotional expression as well as the attempted repression of thoughts, feelings, and sensations associated with emotional experience. Ironically, such emotional inhibition positively correlates with negative thoughts, negative affect, and psychological distress including depression and anxiety. A pattern of emotional inhibition as an adult also mediated the relationship between negative emotion socialization experiences in childhood and adult psychological distress (Krause et al., 2003). The present research expanded on these findings by demonstrating that emotional inhibition also mediated the relationship between experiences of child psychological maltreatment and adult intimate partner victimization. Thus, while suppressing emotional expression and experience may enable a child to feel less overwhelmed in a stressful environment, this emotional inhibition may have negative long-term consequences for the adult.

By demonstrating how survivors of child psychological maltreatment may become adult victims and/or perpetrators of aggression, the present study further exemplifies the importance of studying intimate partner violence as a problem that often involves mutual infliction of aggression (Bradbury & Lawrence, 1999; DiLillo et al., 2001; Stets & Straus, 1989). Benjamin (2003) maintains that people tend to repeat abusive situations because they have not yet let go of the wish that an important other who has hurt them will someday meet their needs. In different ways, survivors of abuse may exhibit relational difficulties in an attempt to provide a "gift of love" to their childhood aggressor. First, through recapitulation, a survivor of abuse may find him/herself in future abusive relationships, essentially behaving as if the original perpetrator is still there and in control. A survivor of child abuse may thus find that being intimate with an abusive partner is familiar and may even be drawn (albeit subconsciously) to such relationships in an attempt to work through prior abusive relationships. Sadly, some people who have been interpersonally betrayed may also come to believe that they are not worthy or capable of being in a mutually respectful relationship (Jordan, Walker, & Hartling, 2004).

Another mechanism by which survivors of child abuse may attempt to resolve childhood conflict is by identification with the aggressor, and through this mechanism survivors of child abuse may become abusive themselves (Benjamin, 2003). Also, through social learning, the patterns of interpersonal contempt, ridicule, aggression and coercion that have been observed in the parents can be imitated and result in similar patterns of relating to intimate partners (Patterson, 1982). These patterns can be stored as interpersonal scripts in the form of schemas and become activated in situations evocative of the setting in which they were learned (Baldwin, 1992). Thus, romantic relationships, with their focus on intimacy, affection, and care giving, might be prime targets for such interpersonal expectancies to be enacted.

In the present study, schemas of mistrust, entitlement, emotional inhibition, and insufficient self-control all emerged as partial mediators of the association between experiences of child psychological maltreatment and self-reported perpetration of adult interpersonal aggression. Survivors of child psychological maltreatment who expected others to mistreat them were more susceptible to committing aggressive acts in their adult relationships. Further research is needed to clarify the frequency with which such acts tend to be initiated by the survivors, or are instead self-defense responses to perceived or actual victimization. In addition, our results indicate that survivors who repeatedly deny their own emotional expression may be likely to themselves become perpetrators of aggression. It seems that for some, consistently refraining from expressing one's needs is apt to lead to a pent-up frustration of those needs, ultimately culminating in an explosion of aggression.

The two schemas that were uniquely associated with perpetration of aggression, and not with victimization experiences, were particularly informative in this regard. Both of these schemas, insufficient self-control and entitlement, comprise the domain of impaired limits articulated by Young and colleagues (2003). The schema of insufficient self-control reflects a negative sense of one's own ability to tolerate frustration. From the perspective of attachment theory, children rely on their parents for help in regulating their arousal (Bowlby, 1982). However, when a child's parents are frequently emotionally abusive, the child's arousal level may be chronically heightened, leading to difficulties developing effective emotion regulation strategies (Gunnar, Brodersen, Nachmias, Buss, & Rigatuso, 1996; Yates, 2007). As young adults, survivors of such abuse may have particular difficulty regulating their emotions in conflict situations and resort to hostile, negative, and abusive patterns of responding.

Finally, the schema of entitlement denotes the belief that one deserves special privileges, and it is often associated with a disregard for others' needs and feelings. Individuals with feelings of entitlement are often preoccupied with asserting and defending their rights and collecting on debts they believe are owed to them (Bishop & Lane, 2002;

Exline, Baumeister, Bushman, Campbell, & Finkel, 2004). Feelings of entitlement are, thus, particularly likely to translate into interpersonal expectations since these feelings pertain to one's assumptions about how other people should treat the self (Exline et al., 2004). Since the special treatment that is expected is often not forthcoming, relational struggles are likely to ensue (Benjamin, 2003). A person who endorses a schema of entitlement may expect to get what he or she wants from a partner, and be easily offended, quick to anger, and vengeful if this does not occur. Such a profile has been linked to a propensity towards sexual aggression in situations where sexual acquiescence has been expected (Bushman, Bonacci, van Dijk, & Baumeister, 2003). Prior research has also documented that there is a defensive aspect to entitlement (Bishop & Lane, 2002). The entitled person can be determined to assert his or her rights in an effort to maintain a fragile sense of self-esteem and to save face (Bushman et al., 2003; Bushman & Baumeister, 1998).

Cloitre and colleagues (2002) suggest that reducing susceptibility to later revictimization in child abuse survivors may necessitate changing existing relational schemas. This study provides further support that this may be needed, especially for those who are at risk of becoming victims or perpetrators of relationship aggression. Exploration of individuals' relationship histories, both historically and contemporaneously, may provide important clues regarding the nature of interpersonal scripts that have been learned regarding patterns of relating to an intimate partner. Such a detailed understanding of the person's "expectations about what behaviors tend to be followed by what responses" could provide a more effective means of intervening with individuals at risk for experiencing relationship aggression (Baldwin, 1992, p. 468). Individuals with histories of child psychological maltreatment have been exposed to many negative interpersonal dynamics in which issues of power, control, and conflict management have been poorly managed (DiLillo et al., 2001). Such survivors need opportunities, both within subsequent interpersonal relationships, and if needed, in therapy, to observe positive and effective forms of interpersonal relating during high conflict or stressful situations (DiLillo et al., 2001). The experience of shame and powerlessness that often accompanies psychological abuse is also a very important, but neglected, area and one that is likely to significantly impact emotional reactivity (either in terms of inhibition or loss of control of emotion) to perceived threats to self-esteem and self-worth (Harper, Austin, Cercone, & Arias, 2005). Since schemas may be a critical pathway through which early abusive experiences are expressed, further research exploring how shame and low self-worth are reflected in interpersonal schemas such as mistrust, self-sacrifice, emotional inhibition, insufficient self-control, or entitlement, and how such schemas guide subsequent behavior in romantic relationships is needed. Such information will likely enrich our understanding of how to design effective intervention programs for young adults at risk for experiencing relationship aggression.

LIMITATIONS

Several limitations of the current investigation should be noted. The results, although representing an important exploratory study in this area, need to be interpreted with caution. First, the participants were all American college students and the majority of them were also Caucasian. Consequently, the findings obtained may not generalize to community samples or individuals of other socioeconomic statuses, educational levels, or cultural backgrounds. Second, reliance on retrospective self-report data may have introduced the possibility of method variance that could have influenced the participants' response set across the questionnaires. Individuals who reported difficulty on one measure may have been more likely to do so across measures, thus inflating the degree of relationship across these areas. Third, concerns about social desirability may have impacted participants' willingness to acknowledge victimization or perpetration experiences, and so these experiences may have been under-reported. However, across this relatively large sample, there was a continuous distribution of responses, suggesting a good range of scores on each measure. We attempted to minimize concerns about child abuse definitions by incorporating a well-validated and comprehensive measure of child maltreatment that included 82 behaviorally anchored items. Use of this measure allowed us to examine the continuum of psychologically abusive childhood experiences, rather than having to make a decision about a specific cutoff score demarcating abuse. The measures of interpersonal schemas, dating abuse, and aggression were selected because they were well-standardized measures. Finally, the correlational design of the study limited inferences about causal relationships, leaving other interpretations of the data open to possibility. Future studies need to include more diverse populations, alternative methods of assessment such as interviewing, and if possible, prospective and qualitative research designs.

CONCLUSIONS

This study represents an initial attempt to explore factors that might serve as important mediators of the relationship between later perpetration and/or revictimization experiences in both male and female child abuse survivors. Our findings provide a unique window into the relational expectations that some survivors of child abuse hold and suggest that it is advantageous for future research on intimate partner violence to be driven by theory on interpersonal schemas, as such studies are apt to lead us to answers about the circumstances under which intimate partner aggression is probable and amenable to intervention. Children who experience repeated invalidation of their emotions, and who come to believe that they are worthless except to meet others' needs, are susceptible to subsequent unhealthy relationships in adulthood that may even be characterized by aggression. The results of this study indicate that the survivors who are most vulnerable to experiencing abusive adult relationships are those who hold interpersonal schemas of others as likely to perpetrate abuse, or who believe that they must prioritize others' needs above their own. Consistently suppressing one's own expression of emotions is also apt to increase the likelihood that a survivor of child psychological abuse will be revictimized as an adult, or will eventually explode by perpetrating interpersonally aggressive acts. In addition, abuse survivors who have little confidence in their own ability to tolerate frustration, or who have a fragile self-esteem that presents itself as a sense of entitlement, are at risk for responding to interpersonal conflict with aggression. Our results reiterate the importance of intervening early with child abuse survivors in order to address the component of psychological abuse that they have endured in a manner that affords survivors the opportunity to alter existing relational schemas. It is intuitive that for child abuse survivors, the experience of trustworthy, mutually respectful relationships is the best antidote to the perpetuation of a cycle of interpersonal aggression.

REFERENCES

Arata, C. M. (2002). Child sexual abuse and sexual revictimization. *Clinical Psychology Science and Practice, 9*, 135-164.

Baldwin, M. W. (1992). Relational schemas and the processing of social information. *Psychological Bulletin, 112*, 461-484.

Baron, R. M., & Kenny, D. A. (1986). The moderator-mediator variable distinction in social psychological research: Conceptual, strategic, and statistical considerations. *Journal of Personality and Social Psychology, 51*, 1173-1182.

Bellow, S. M., Boris, N. W., Larrieu, J. A., Lewis, M. L., & Elliot, A. (2005). Conceptual and clinical dilemmas in defining and assessing role reversal in young child-caregiver relationships. *Journal of Emotional Abuse, 5*, 43-66.

Benjamin, L. S. (2003). *Interpersonal reconstructive therapy: Promoting change in nonresponders.* New York: The Guilford Press.

Bensley, L., Van Eenwyk, J., & Simmons, K. W. (2003). Childhood family violence history and women's risk for intimate partner violence and poor health. *American Journal of Preventive Medicine, 25*(1), 38-44.

Bierer, L. M., Yehuda, R. L., Schmeidler, J., Mitropoulou, V., New, A. S., Silverman, J. M. et al. (2003). Abuse and neglect in childhood: Relationship to personality disorder diagnoses. *CNS Spectrums, 8*, 737-740, 749-754.

Bifulco, A., Moran, P. M., Baines, R., Bunn, A., & Stanford, K. (2002). Exploring psychological abuse in childhood: II. Association with other abuse and adult clinical depression. *Bulletin of the Menninger Clinic, 66*, 241-258.

Bishop, J., & Lane, R. C. (2002). The dynamics and dangers of entitlement. *Psychoanalytic Psychology, 19*, 739-758.

Bowlby, J. (1982). *Attachment and loss: Vol. 1. Attachment* (2nd ed.). New York: Basic Books.

Bradbury, T. N., & Lawrence, E. (1999). Physical aggression and the longitudinal course of newlywed marriage. In X. B. Arriaga & S. Oskamp (Eds.), *Violence in intimate relationships* (pp. 181-202). Thousand Oaks, CA: Sage.

Bushman, B. J., Bonacci, A. M., van Dijk, M., & Baumeister, R. F. (2003). Narcissism, sexual refusal, and aggression: Testing a narcissistic reactance model of sexual coercion. *Journal of Personality and Social Psychology, 84*, 1027-1040.

Bushman, B. J., & Baumeister, R. F. (1998). Threatened egotism, narcissism, self-esteem, and direct and displaced aggression: Does self-love or self-hate lead to violence? *Journal of Personality and Social Psychology, 75*, 219-229.

Buss, A. H., & Perry, M. (1992). The aggression questionnaire. *Journal of Personality and Social Psychology, 63*(3), 452-459.

Cicchetti, D., & Toth, S. L. (1995). A developmental psychopathology perspective on child abuse and neglect. *Journal of the Academy of Child and Adolescent Psychiatry, 34*, 541-565.

Cicchetti, D., & Toth, S. L. (2000). Developmental processes in maltreated children. In D. J. Hansen (Ed.), *Nebraska symposium on motivation: Child maltreatment* (Vol. 46, pp. 85-160). Lincoln, NE: University of Nebraska Press.

Cloitre, M., Cohen, L. R., & Scarvalone, P. (2002). Understanding revictimization among childhood sexual abuse survivors: An interpersonal schema approach. *Journal of Cognitive Psychotherapy: An International Quarterly, 16*(1), 91-111.

Collins, N. L., Guichard, A. C., Ford, M. B., & Feeney, B. C. (2004). Working models of attachment: New developments and emerging themes. In W. S. Rholes & J. A. Simpson (Eds.), *Adult attachment: Theory, research and clinical implications* (pp. 196-239). New York: Guilford Press.

Davis, J. L., Petretic-Jackson, P. A., & Ting, L. (2001). Intimacy dysfunction and trauma symptomatology: Long-term correlates of different types of child abuse. *Journal of Traumatic Stress, 14*(1), 63-79.

DiLillo, D., Giuffre, D., Tremblay, G. C., & Peterson, L. (2001). A closer look at the nature of intimate partner violence reported by women with a history of child sexual abuse. *Journal of Interpersonal Violence, 16*(2), 116-132.

Drapeau, M., & Perry, J. C. (2004). Childhood trauma and adult interpersonal functioning: A study using the Core Conflictual Relationship Theme Method (CCRT). *Child Abuse and Neglect, 28*, 1049-1066.

Ehrensaft, M. K., Cohen, P., Brown, J., Smailes, E., Chen, H., & Johnson, J.G. (2003). Intergenerational transmission of partner violence: A 20-year prospective study. *Journal of Consulting and Clinical Psychology, 71*, 741-753.

Exline, J. J., Baumeister, R. F., Bushman, B. J., Campbell, W. K., & Finkel, E. J. (2004). Too proud to let go: Narcissistic entitlement as a barrier to forgiveness. *Journal of Personality and Social Psychology, 87*, 894-912.

Fortin, A., & Chamberland, C. (1995). Preventing the psychological maltreatment of children. *Journal of Interpersonal Violence, 10*(3), 275-295.

Gibb, B. E., Alloy, L. B., Abramson, L. Y., Rose, D. T., Whitehouse, W. G., Donovan, P. et al. (2001). History of childhood maltreatment, negative cognitive styles, and episodes of depression in adulthood. *Cognitive Therapy and Research, 25*(4), 425-446.

Glaser, D. (2002). Emotional abuse and neglect (psychological maltreatment): A conceptual framework. *Child Abuse and Neglect, 26*, 697-714.

Gunnar, M. R., Brodersen, L., Nachmias, M., Buss, K., & Rigatuso, J. (1996). Stress reactivity and attachment security. *Developmental Psychobiology, 29*, 191-204.

Hamarman, S., & Bernet, W. (2000). Evaluating and reporting emotional abuse in children: Parent-based, action-based focus aids in clinical decision-making. *Journal of American Academy of Child and Adolescent Psychiatry, 39*(7), 928-930.

Harper, F. W. K., Austin, A. G., Cercone, J. J., & Arias, I. (2005). The role of shame, anger, and affect regulation in men's perpetration of psychological abuse in dating relationships. *Journal of Interpersonal Violence, 20*(12), 1648-1662.

Harris, A. E., & Curtin, L. (2002). Parental perceptions, early maladaptive schemas, and depressive symptoms in young adults. *Cognitive Therapy and Research, 26*(3), 405-416.

Higgins, D. J., & McCabe, M. P. (2000). Relationships between different types of maltreatment during childhood and adjustment in adulthood. *Child Maltreatment, 5*, 261-272.

Higgins, D. J., & McCabe, M. P. (2001). Multiple forms of child abuse and neglect: Adult retrospective reports. *Aggression and Violent Behavior, 6*, 547-578.

Hodgins, D. C., Maticka-Tyndale, E., El-Guebaly, N., & West, M. (1993). The CAST-6: Development of a short-form of the children of alcoholics screening test. *Addictive Behaviors, 18*, 337-345.

Jordan, J. V., Walker, M., & Hartling, L. M. (2004). *The complexity of connection.* New York: Guilford Press.

Kent, A., & Waller, G. (2000). Childhood emotional abuse and eating psychopathology. *Clinical Psychology Review, 20*, 887-903.

Koss, M., & Gidycz, C. (1982). Sexual experiences survey: A research instrument. *Journal of Consulting and Clinical Psychology, 50*(3), 455-457.

Krause, E. D., Mendelson, T., & Lynch, T. R. (2003). Childhood emotional invalidation and adult psychological distress: The mediating role of emotional inhibition. *Child Abuse and Neglect, 27*, 199-213.

Lang, A. J., Stein M. B., Kennedy, C. M., & Foy, D. W. (2004). Adult psychopathology and intimate partner violence among survivors of childhood maltreatment. *Journal of Interpersonal Violence, 19*, 1102-1118.

Linder, J. R., & Collins, W. A. (2005). Parent and peer predictors of physical aggression and conflict management in romantic relationships in early adulthood. *Journal of Family Psychology, 19*(2), 252-262.

Manly, J. T., Kim, J. E., Rogosch, F. A., & Cicchetti, D. (2001). Dimensions of child maltreatment and children's adjustment: Contributions of developmental timing and subtype. *Development and Psychopathology, 13*, 759-782.

McGee, R. A., Wolfe, D. A., & Wilson, S. K. (1997). Multiple maltreatment experiences and adolescent behavior problems: Adolescents' perspectives. *Development and Psychopathology, 9*, 131-149.

Messman-Moore, T. L., & Long, P. J. (2003). The role of childhood sexual abuse sequelae in sexual revictimization: An empirical review and theoretical reformulation. *Clinical Psychology Review, 23*, 537-571.

Newton, T. L., & Weigel, R. A. (2007). Cardiovascular correlates of mistreatment in healthy adults. *Journal of Emotional Abuse 7*(2), 35-58.

Patterson, G. R. (1982). *Coercive family process.* Eugene, OR: Castalia.

Sanders, B., and Becker-Lausen, E. (1995). The measurement of psychological maltreatment: Early data on the child abuse and trauma scale. *Child Abuse and Neglect, 19*(3), 315-323.

Schneider, M. W., Ross, A., Graham, J. C., & Zielinski, A. (2005). Do allegations of emotional maltreatment predict developmental outcomes beyond that of other forms of maltreatment? *Child Abuse and Neglect, 29*, 513-532.

Stets, J. E., & Straus, M. A. (1989). The marriage license as a hitting license: A comparison of assaults in dating, cohabitating, and married couples. *Journal of Family Violence, 4*, 161-180.

Stevens, J. P. (2002). *Applied multivariate statistics for the social sciences* (4th ed.). Mahwah, NJ: Lawrence Erlbaum Associates.

Stith, S. M., Rosen, K. H., Middleton, K. A., Busch, A. L., Lundeberg, K., & Carlton, R. P. (2000). The intergenerational transmission of spouse abuse: A meta-analysis. *Journal of Marriage and the Family, 62*, 640-654.

Straus, M. A., Gelles, R. J., & Steinmetz, S. K. (1980). *Behind closed doors: Violence in the American family.* New York: Anchor.

Walter, H. W., & McIntosh, S. R. (1981). The assessment of spouse abuse: Two quantifiable dimensions. *Journal of Marriage and the Family, 43*(4), 873-888.

Whitfield, C. L., Anda, R. F., Dube, S. R., & Felitti, V. H. (2003). Violent childhood experiences and the risk of intimate partner violence in adults. *Journal of Interpersonal Violence, 18*, 166-185.

Yates, T. M. (2007). The developmental consequences of child emotional abuse: A neurodevelopmental perspective. *Journal of Emotional Abuse 7*(2), 9-34.

Young, J. E. (1999). *Cognitive therapy for personality disorders: A schema-focused approach* (3rd edition). Sarasota, FL: Professional Resource Press.
Young, J. E., Klosko, J. S., & Weishaar, M. E. (2003). *Schema therapy: A practitioner's guide.* New York: The Guilford Press.

doi:10.1300/J135v07n02_06

Childhood Psychological Maltreatment and Quality of Marriage: The Mediating Role of Psychological Distress

Andrea R. Perry
David DiLillo
James Peugh

SUMMARY. This study examined the role of adult psychological distress in mediating associations between childhood psychological maltreatment and marital satisfaction in a sample of 65 newlywed couples. Results indicated that a significant linkage between psychological maltreatment (including emotional abuse and emotional neglect) and marital satisfaction was eliminated when accounting for global psychological distress, hostility, and depression in the overall sample. These findings were moderated by gender, such that for men, the long-term correlates of emotional abuse were mediated by broad psychological distress and paranoia. Conversely, for women, relations between emotional abuse and emotional neglect and later marital satisfaction were mediated by obsessive-compulsive tendencies and hostility. The implications of these results for future research and clinical work will be discussed. doi:10.1300/J135v07n02_07 *[Article copies available for a fee from The Haworth Document Delivery Service: 1-800-HAWORTH. E-mail address:*

Address correspondence to: Andrea R. Perry, MA, 238 Burnett Hall, Lincoln, NE 68588-0308 (E-mail: andreaperry1@yahoo.com).

[Haworth co-indexing entry note]: "Childhood Psychological Maltreatment and Quality of Marriage: The Mediating Role of Psychological Distress." Perry, Andrea R., David DiLillo, and James Peugh. Co-published simultaneously in *Journal of Emotional Abuse* (The Haworth Maltreatment & Trauma Press, an imprint of The Haworth Press, Inc.) Vol. 7, No. 2, 2007, pp. 117-142; and: *Childhood Emotional Abuse: Mediating and Moderating Processes Affecting Long-Term Impact* (ed: Margaret O'Dougherty Wright) The Haworth Maltreatment & Trauma Press, an imprint of The Haworth Press, Inc., 2007, pp. 117-142. Single or multiple copies of this article are available for a fee from The Haworth Document Delivery Service [1-800-HAWORTH, 9:00 a.m. - 5:00 p.m. (EST). E-mail address: docdelivery@haworthpress.com].

Available online at http://jea.haworthpress.com

doi:10.1300/J135v07n02_07

KEYWORDS. Psychological maltreatment, emotional abuse, child maltreatment, long-term effects, psychological functioning, marital satisfaction

INTRODUCTION

Until recently, the psychological maltreatment of children has been largely overlooked in the empirical literature and sometimes considered to be only a "side effect" of physical and sexual abuse (Barnett, Miller-Perrin, & Perrin, 1997, p. 120; Hart, Brassard, & Karlson, 1996). As many have contended, the slower emergence of psychological maltreatment as a topic of study may be due, in part, to challenges defining this form of abuse (e.g., Barnett et al., 1997; Claussen & Crittenden, 1991; Fortin & Chamberland, 1995; Hart et al., 1996; Hart, Brassard, Binggeli, & Davidson, 2002; O'Hagan, 1995). For example, unlike physical and sexual abuse, which can be characterized by a discrete set of acts, psychological maltreatment has typically been viewed as comprising a wider range of sometimes subtle caregiver behaviors.

Psychological maltreatment also may reflect a less visible yet enduring condition within the family system (Fortin & Chamberland, 1995; O'Hagan, 1995), as opposed to sexual or physical abuse, which can occur only intermittently and are more likely to come to the attention of outside observers. Further contributing to these definitional ambiguities is the fact that certain questionable tactics (e.g., yelling, emotional withdrawal) occur at some point in the majority of parent-child dyads, making it difficult to distinguish between negative, yet sub-threshold interactions and those that cross the blurry line into abuse (Barnett et al., 1997; Claussen & Crittenden, 1991; Glaser, 2002; O'Hagan, 1995; Straus & Field, 2003; Twaite & Rodriguez-Srednicki, 2004; Vissing, Straus, Gelles, & Harrop, 1991).

Regardless of the definition used, research has shown that childhood psychological maltreatment is disturbingly common (see Barnett et al., 1997; Hart & Brassard, 1987; Hart et al., 2002). For example, adult retrospective reports indicate that the prevalence of psychological maltreatment ranges from 5.6% to 34.8%, depending on the type of sample used (Edwards, Holden, Felitti, & Anda, 2003; Moeller, Bachmann, & Moeller, 1993; Mullen, Martin, Anderson, Romans, & Herbison, 1996).

When distinguishing between emotionally abusive versus neglectful acts, researchers have reported that emotional abuse ranges from 12.1% to 45.9% and that emotional neglect ranges from 5.1% to 83.4% (Medrano, Zule, Hatch, & Desmond, 1999; Scher, Forde, McQuaid, & Stein, 2004; Spertus, Yehuda, Wong, Halligan, & Seremetis, 2003). In addition to being common, psychological maltreatment frequently co-occurs with, and is exacerbated by, other forms of child maltreatment (e.g., Claussen & Crittenden, 1991; Edwards et al., 2003; Glaser, 2002). In fact, psychological maltreatment has been labeled by some as the "core issue" (Claussen & Crittenden, 1991; Hart & Brassard, 1987, p. 161) and "unifying concept . . . of child abuse and neglect" (Barnett et al., 1997; Hart et al., 1996; Hart et al., 2002, p. 79).

ASSOCIATIONS BETWEEN PSYCHOLOGICAL MALTREATMENT AND MENTAL HEALTH FUNCTIONING

Psychological maltreatment has been linked to a range of long-term mental health difficulties. For example, a history of psychological maltreatment has been associated with general psychological distress (Wark, Kruczek, & Boley, 2003), diminished self-esteem (Briere & Runtz, 1990; Mullen et al., 1996; Twaite & Rodriguez-Srednicki, 2004), internalized shame (Twaite & Rodriguez-Srednicki, 2004), emotional inhibition (including suppressed/withheld thoughts, avoidant coping styles, and ambivalence regarding emotional expression; Krause, Mendelson, & Lynch, 2003), and a negative cognitive style (Gibb, 2002). Linkages also have been found for other internalizing difficulties, such as depression (Spertus et al., 2003), anxiety (Briere & Runtz, 1988; Spertus et al., 2003), dissociation (Briere & Runtz, 1988), and posttraumatic stress symptomatology (Spertus et al., 2003), as well as externalizing problems, including physically aggressive behaviors and delinquency (Vissing et al., 1991), suicidal ideation (Gibb et al., 2001; Mullen et al., 1996), substance use (Moran, Vuchinich, & Hall, 2004), and other risky health behaviors such as not wearing a seatbelt and engaging in sexual intercourse at a younger age (Rodgers et al., 2004).

Associations Between Psychological Maltreatment and Interpersonal Functioning

In the realm of adult interpersonal functioning, a range of proximal factors such as conflict resolution, interpartner communication, and psychological functioning is associated with satisfaction and distress in romantic dyads (Davila & Bradbury, 1998; Kurdek, 1995; Rogge & Bradbury, 1999). More recently, researchers have begun to highlight the effects of more distal events, such as sexual abuse and exposure to domestic violence, on long-term dyadic functioning (Colman & Widom, 2004; DiLillo & Long, 1999; Halford, Sanders, & Behrens, 2000). Consistent with these findings, it is plausible that psychological maltreatment may impede the development of satisfying relationships in adulthood (Davis, Petretic-Jackson, & Ting, 2001). In fact, in contrast to other abuse types, psychological maltreatment may be particularly harmful because it involves a parent or caregiver *directly* imparting negative messages to the childmessages that often highlight the youth' perceived inadequacies or failures (e.g., Gibb, Alloy, Abramson, & Marx, 2003; Spertus et al., 2003; Twaite & Rodriguez-Srednicki, 2004). These often manipulative messages leave little room for interpretation on the part of the child and render it difficult for victims to learn appropriate ways to interpret and express emotions and engage in adaptive self-care (Gibb, 2002; O'Hagan, 1995; Spertus et al., 2003). From a social learning perspective, these messages may be internalized by the child and extended into adulthood in the form of negative schemas about self, others, and the world (Hart & Brassard, 1987; Twaite & Rodriguez-Srednicki, 2004). Similarly, attachment theorists have posited that early parental messages contribute to a core belief system–or interpersonal template–by which child victims will come to view themselves and others, including romantic partners (Collins, Guichard, Ford, & Feeney, 2004; Hart et al., 2002; Thomas, 2003; Thompson, Laible, & Ontai, 2003; Twaite & Rodriguez-Srednicki, 2004).

Consistent with these views, research has begun to show that psychological maltreatment is in fact associated with interpersonal consequences across the lifespan. Specifically, early psychological maltreatment can disrupt the development of secure attachment relationships with caregivers, contributing to displays of avoidance and dependency among maltreated children (e.g., Barnett et al., 1997; Egeland, 1991; Glaser, 2002; Hart et al., 1996), and may adversely impact child and adolescent peer relationships. For instance, psychological maltreatment is associated with withdrawal from peers, anxiety surrounding relationships (such as worries about being judged), aggression directed at other children and adolescents, and difficulty establishing and maintaining friendships (Barnett et al., 1997; Bolger & Patterson, 2001; Fortin & Chamberland, 1995; Glaser, 2002; Hart et al., 1996; Kairys, Johnson, & the Committee on Child Abuse and Neglect, 2002; Vissing et al., 1991). Similarly, adults with a history of psychological maltreatment report increased loneliness and isolation from relationships (Loos & Alexander, 1997), decreased trust in and closeness to their romantic partners (Twaite & Rodriguez-Srednicki, 2004), and heightened interpersonal sensitivity (Briere & Runtz, 1988), and they may hold beliefs that their spouse is excessively intrusive and uncaring (Mullen et al., 1996). In addition, psychological maltreatment, either alone or in combination with other maltreatment, has also been linked to sexual difficulties (Mullen et al., 1996), fear associated with intimacy (Davis et al., 2001), and eventual marital termination (Mullen et al., 1996).

Associations Between Psychological and Interpersonal Functioning

As described, psychological maltreatment is linked to lasting difficulties in the realms of mental health and relationship functioning. In addition, there is evidence from couples literature that individual psychological functioning and dyadic adjustment are highly interrelated (e.g., Davila & Bradbury, 1998; Fruzzetti, 1996; Prince & Jacobson, 1995). For example, greater depression and anxiety symptoms have been linked to lower marital satisfaction in community couples (Whisman, Uebelacker, & Weinstock, 2004), an association that may be bidirectional in nature (Davila & Bradbury, 1998; Davila, Bradbury, Cohan, & Tochluk, 1997). Different patterns also have emerged for men and women. For instance, it appears that husbands' depressive symptoms are causally related to decreased marital satisfaction. However, for wives, heightened marital dysfunction seems to lead to impaired mental health functioning (Fincham, Beach, Harold, & Osborne, 1997). In light of strong connections between adults' mental health and interpersonal functioning, it is not surprising that, even after controlling for marital satisfaction and the affective state of one's spouse, men's and women's dysphoric symptoms have been found to adversely impact couple interactions (e.g., utilization of less effective conflict resolution tactics; Du Rocher Schudlich, Papp, & Cummings, 2004).

Present Study: Evaluating Psychological Functioning as a Mediator

Although several studies have underscored the long-term intrapersonal and interpersonal correlates of psychological maltreatment, we are aware of no investigations that have simultaneously examined associations among all three of these constructs. When considering possible relations among these variables, prior research showing that psychological maltreatment impinges on both psychological and interpersonal difficulties, as well as findings that individual distress often leads to dyadic (including marital) problems, suggests that adult psychological symptoms may mediate associations between psychological maltreatment history and later relationship quality. This possibility is consistent with findings that cumulative maltreatment history operates through individual distress to impact relationship functioning among unmarried college students (DiLillo, Lewis, & DiLoreto-Colgan, in press). Similarly, here it was expected that associations between early psychological maltreatment, including both abuse and neglect, and adult relationship quality would be mediated by psychological distress in a sample of randomly recruited newlywed couples. Further, based on previously cited work discussing the potency of psychological maltreatment relative to other abuse types (e.g., Fortin & Chamberland, 1995; Glaser, 2002; Hart & Brassard, 1987; Hart et al., 2002), psychological maltreatment was expected to maintain these associations even after controlling for other forms of child maltreatment, including sexual abuse, physical abuse, and physical neglect. Finally, based on findings that the relationship between mental health symptoms and marital satisfaction differs for men and women (Fincham et al., 1997), these associations were examined not only for the overall sample but also separately for husbands and wives.

METHOD

Participants

Participants were 65 newlywed couples (N = 130 participants) recruited from publicly available marriage license records in Lancaster County, Nebraska. Couples qualified as newlyweds if they had been married one year or less at the time they were recruited to participate in the study; they were also required to be at least 19 years of age, which is the age of majority in the state of Nebraska. In the current study, couples had been married on average 11.31 months (SD = .54, range = 11 to 14 months). Participants ages ranged from 21 to 85 (M = 32.31, SD = 10.73). Regarding ethnicity, 93% were European American, 3% African American, 2.3% Hispanic American, .8% Asian American, and .8% Native American. Reports of the current household income were as follows: $20,000 or less = 14.1%; $21,000 to 30,000 = 14.1%; $31,000 to 40,000 = 14.1%; $41,000 to 50,000 = 13.3%; $51,000 to 60,000 = 17%;

$61,000 to 70,000 = 5.2%; $71,000 to 80,000 = 8.1%; $81,000 to 90,000 = 3.0%, $91,000 to 100,000 = 2.2%, and greater than $100,000 = 6.0%). Finally, although the majority of participants were in their first marriage, 18.6% of participants indicated that they had at least one previous marriage.

Measures

Brief Symptom Inventory (BSI; Derogatis, 1993). The BSI, which is comprised of 53 self-report items, assesses psychopathology and psychological distress across nine Primary Symptom Dimensions (i.e., Somatization, Obsessive-Compulsive, Interpersonal Sensitivity, Depression, Anxiety, Hostility, Phobic Anxiety, Paranoid Ideation, and Psychoticism) and three Global Indices (i.e., Global Severity Index, Positive Symptom Distress Index, and Positive Symptom Total; Derogatis, 1993, 1994; Derogatis & Melisaratos, 1983). In the current study, analyses included each of the Primary Symptom Dimensions as well as the Global Severity Index (referred to henceforth as the BSI Total), which measures overall levels of psychological distress. Participants rated each question based on "how much that problem has distressed or bothered [them] during the past 7 days including today" on a Likert scale (0 = *not at all*, 1 = *a little bit*, 2 = *moderately*, 3 = *quite a bit*, 4 = *extremely*). The types of difficulties measured were, for example, nervousness or shakiness inside, feeling easily annoyed or irritated, feeling lonely, not feeling close to others, and trouble concentrating (Derogatis & Melisaratos, 1983).

The psychometric properties of the BSI have been well documented. BSI subscales are strongly correlated to parallel constructs on the SCL-90, with ranges from .92 to .99 (Derogatis, 1994). Internal consistency estimates for BSI subscales range from .64 to .87 in a large sample of college students in outpatient therapy (Hayes, 1997), from .71 to .85 among outpatient psychiatric clients (Derogatis & Melisaratos, 1983), from .75 to .89 in a group of psychiatric in- and outpatients (Boulet & Boss, 1991), and from .60 to .83 in a similar community sample of newlywed couples (DiLillo, 2006). In addition, among a non-patient normative sample, test-retest reliability with a two-week testing interval ranged from .68 to .91 across the nine Primary Symptom dimensions and .90 on the Global Symptom Index (Derogatis & Melisaratos, 1983).

Childhood Trauma Questionnaire (CTQ; Bernstein & Fink, 1998). The CTQ is a 28-item self-report questionnaire designed to assess adolescents' and adults' retrospective reports of child maltreatment, including emotional abuse, emotional neglect, sexual abuse, physical abuse, and physical neglect. Five questions are included for each form of child maltreatment. Participants indicate whether they experienced certain events while growing up on a scale from 1 = *never true* to 5 = *very often true*. For instance, the emotional abuse scale, which measures "verbal assaults on a child's sense of worth or well-being, or any humiliating, demeaning, or threatening behavior directed toward a child by an older person," encompasses questions such as whether a participant recalls being called names (e.g., "stupid," "lazy," or "ugly" or whether a participant believes that he or she was emotionally abused. Similarly, in order to ascertain emotionally neglectful experiences, defined as "the failure of caretakers to provide a child's basic psychological and emotional needs, such as love, encouragement, belonging, and support," participants report, for example, whether there was someone in their family who helped them feel important or special (Bernstein & Fink, 1998, p. 2).

One advantage of the CTQ is that it produces continuous rather than simply dichotomous scores for each type of maltreatment, with higher scores indicating greater levels of that form of abuse. These continuous scores can be translated into an abuse severity classification (i.e., *None* or *Minimal*, *Low* or *Moderate*, *Moderate* or *Severe*, and *Severe* or *Extreme*). Utilizing Receiver Operating Characteristic (ROC) analysis, Bernstein and Fink (1998) validated these severity classifications, or cut scores, by interviewing a sample of HMO members about their trauma history and comparing the interview data to participants' CTQ responses. When generating the cut scores, the authors sought to maximize the inclusion of low severity cases (including 80% of these cases) while keeping false positives to a rate of 20% or less.

The abuse subtype scores have been shown to have excellent psychometric properties, including high internal consistency across a variety of inpatient, outpatient, and student populations (emotional abuse = .83 – .94; emotional neglect = .81 – .93) and strong test-retest reliability with, on average, a 3.6 month test interval (emotional abuse = .80, emotional neglect = .81; Bernstein & Fink, 1998). Other researchers have corroborated these findings. For example, in a large community sample, internal consistency for emotional abuse and emotional neglect has been reported as .83 and .85, respectively (Scher, Stein, Asmundson, McCreary, & Forde, 2001), and test-retest reliability in a college student sample was .96 for emotional abuse and .97 for emotional neglect after an 8-10 week testing interval (Paivio & Cramer,

2004). Finally, confirmatory factor analyses conducted for each type of maltreatment have revealed that the five CTQ subscales "hang" together across diverse samples (Bernstein & Fink, 1998; Scher et al., 2001).

Quality Marriage Index (QMI; Norton, 1983). The QMI is a six-item self-report scale designed to measure marital satisfaction by inquiring about the stability and strength of the marital relationship. Participants chose answers from five alternatives: *never true, occasionally true, often true, frequently true,* and *always true* on a scale of 1 to 5. An additional question asked participants to rate the degree of their overall happiness within the marriage, ranging from 1 = *very unhappy* to 7 = *very happy*. Higher scores on the QMI indicated higher marital satisfaction, whereas lower scores corresponded with lower satisfaction. Recent studies have documented excellent internal reliability estimates in community-based couples, ranging from .94 (Whisman & Delinsky, 2002) to .97 (Culp & Beach, 1998; Heyman, Sayers, & Bellack, 1994). The QMI also has acceptable discriminant validity, with low correlations emerging between marital satisfaction and many Symptom Checklist 90-Revised mental health symptoms, as well as convergent validity with two other marital functioning measures: the Dyadic Adjustment Scale and the Relationship Satisfaction Questionnaire (Heyman et al., 1994).

Procedure

Couples were identified by public marriage records and were mailed a letter inviting them to participate in a study "exploring the relationship between different childhood experiences and the ways that men and women adapt to their marriages." Consistent with studies utilizing a similar methodology (Davila et al., 1997; Karney et al., 1995; Kurdek, 2002, 2005), approximately 15% of couples agreed to participate. Interested couples came to the university laboratory and completed measures on a computer in separate rooms to ensure privacy. The measures used in this study were part of a larger battery of questionnaires. Prior to participating, couples signed an informed consent form and were assured that they could stop at any time without penalty. A $75 incentive was paid to each couple upon completion of the study. Participants also received a debriefing form after completing the study. The study was approved by the University of Nebraska-Lincoln Institutional Review Board.

RESULTS

Descriptive Characteristics of the Sample

Descriptive statistics for all independent and dependent variables are presented in Table 1. A total of 90.4% of participants reported Quality of Marriage Index total scores falling in the above average range, while only 13 participants had item responses indicative of average or below average marital satisfaction. Brief Symptom Inventory Global Severity Index scores showed that 25 participants (18.5%) reported score elevations indicative of distressed psychological functioning (defined as *T*-scores of 65 or greater). In addition, according to the CTQ cut scores, 46.7% of participants reported experiencing emotional abuse, 74.1% emotional neglect, 34.7% physical abuse, 23.7% physical neglect, and 11.1% sexual abuse.

Variable Relationships and Path Analysis Models

Table 2 lists the results of bivariate correlational analyses between the dependent variable (Quality of Marriage Index scores) and scores

TABLE 1. Descriptive Statistics

	Overall		Females		Males	
Variable	*Mean*	*S.D.*	*Mean*	*S.D.*	*Mean*	*S.D.*
BSI	*N* = 133		*n* = 65		*n* = 65	
Total Score	25.83	24.99	29.22	26.38	22.63	23.63
Psychoticism	3.59	4.48	4.23	4.68	3.05	4.31
Hostility	2.68	2.76	2.83	3.02	2.51	2.41
Anxiety	2.47	3.42	3.03	3.97	1.91	2.76
Somatization	2.68	3.98	3.08	4.39	2.26	3.54
Phobic Anxiety	1.43	2.36	2.02	2.89	0.86	1.53
Paranoid Ideation	3.62	4.27	4.09	4.42	3.18	4.17
Depression	4.31	4.76	5.14	4.88	3.52	4.59
Obsessive-Compulsive	4.56	4.45	4.58	4.52	4.58	4.45
CTQ						
Emotional Abuse	9.32	4.70	9.54	4.84	8.77	4.26
Physical Abuse	7.75	3.90	7.25	3.29	7.92	4.09
Sexual Abuse	6.03	3.20	5.95	2.98	5.55	1.93
Physical Neglect	6.70	2.80	6.28	2.12	6.77	2.96
Emotional Neglect	12.28	3.41	12.08	3.18	12.29	3.53
QMI Total	27.16	5.32	26.66	5.96	27.43	4.64

Note: Five participants were pairwise deleted for failure to indicate their gender.

TABLE 2. Variable Correlations

	Quality of Marriage Index (QMI)		
Variable	Overall	Females	Males
	N = 133	*n = 65*	*n = 65*
BSI			
Total Score	–0.48**	–0.48**	–0.48**
Psychoticism	–0.50**	–0.48**	–0.51**
Hostility	–0.48**	–0.56**	–0.41**
Anxiety	–0.33**	–0.29*	–0.41**
Somatization	–0.29**	–0.24	–0.36**
Phobic Anxiety	–0.20*	–0.16	–0.28*
Paranoid Ideation	–0.39**	–0.49**	–0.25*
Depression	–0.54**	–0.56**	–0.53**
Obsessive-Compulsive	–0.32**	–0.28*	–0.38**
CTQ			
Emotional Abuse	–0.30**	–0.33**	–0.32*
Physical Abuse	–0.16	–0.24	–0.21
Sexual Abuse	–0.06	–0.06	–0.28*
Physical Neglect	–0.01	–0.09	–0.05
Emotional Neglect	–0.24**	–0.33**	–0.22

Note: Five participants were pairwise deleted for failure to indicate their gender.
** = $p < .01$; * = $p < .05$.

for all independent (Childhood Trauma Questionnaire emotional abuse and emotional neglect), mediation (Brief Symptom Inventory total and subscale scores), and covariate (physical abuse, physical neglect, and sexual abuse) variables. Results for the overall sample indicated that all BSI scores (total and subscale scores) were significantly negatively correlated with the QMI; increases in all BSI scores resulted in significant decreases in QMI scores. Results for females indicated that marital satisfaction scores were significantly negatively correlated with: (a) BSI total scores, BSI psychoticism, hostility, anxiety, paranoid ideation, depression, obsessive-compulsive subscale scores, and (b) CTQ emotional abuse and emotional neglect scores. Score increases on those scales were related to significant decreases in QMI scores. Results for males indicated that marital satisfaction scores were significantly negatively correlated with: (a) all BSI scores (total scores and all subscale scores), and (b) CTQ emotional abuse and sexual abuse scores. Score increases on those scales were related to significant QMI score decreases. Table 3 shows the results of bivariate correlational analyses between all child maltreatment subtypes (i.e., sexual abuse, physical abuse, emotional abuse, physical neglect, emotional neglect) for the overall sample and

TABLE 3. Childhood Trauma Questionnaire (CTQ) Variable Intercorrelations

	Overall				
	Emotional Abuse	Physical Abuse	Sexual Abuse	Physical Neglect	Emotional Neglect
Emotional Abuse					
Physical Abuse	.57**				
Sexual Abuse	.54**	.52**			
Physical Neglect	.54**	.59**	.52**		
Emotional Neglect	.62**	.36**	.30**	.51**	
	By Gender				
	Emotional Abuse	Physical Abuse	Sexual Abuse	Physical Neglect	Emotional Neglect
Emotional Abuse					
Physical Abuse	.56**(.59**)				
Sexual Abuse	.49**(.58**)	.52**(.54**)			
Physical Neglect	.60**(.51**)	.60**(.51**)	.54**(.55**)		
Emotional Neglect	.64**(.64**)	.34**(.28**)	0.18(.35**)	.50**(.50**)	

Note: ** = $p < .01$; Male correlations in parentheses.

by gender. With the notable exception of a near-zero correlation between sexual abuse and emotional neglect for females, all maltreatment subtypes were significantly correlated for the overall sample and by gender. Because of the significant correlations among maltreatment subtypes, these variables served as covariates in the path analysis models. Specifically, emotional abuse and emotional neglect each served alternately as independent variables in all direct and mediation path analyses, with the other serving as an additional covariate as shown in Figure 1.

Multicollinearity Assessment

Multicollinearity is a concern in path analysis, especially if the covariates under investigation are cognitive variables (e.g., Stevens, 2002). Two methods available for assessing multicollinearity are

FIGURE 1. Direct and Mediation Path Models

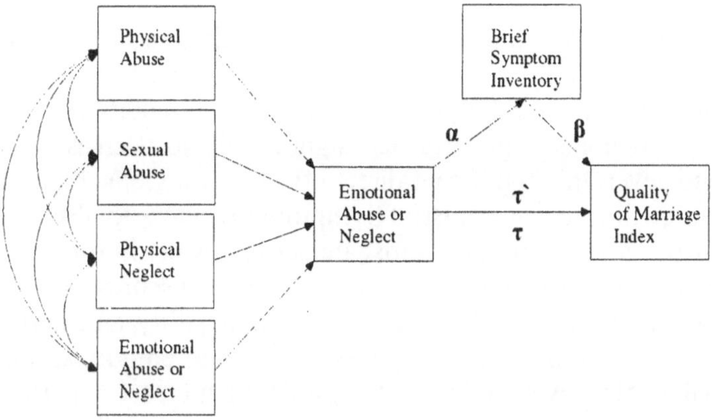

(a) examining the predictor variable correlation matrix, and (b) examining the predictor variable variance inflation factor (VIF) statistics (e.g., Hair, Anderson, Tatham, & Black, 1998; Kline, 2005; Stevens, 2002). As anticipated, a preliminary examination of the correlation matrix and VIF statistics for the predictor variables in this study indicated that multicollinearity (i.e., several bivariate correlation statistics exceeding 0.70 and several predictors with VIF statistics greater than 10) resulted if Brief Symptom Inventory Total scores and BSI subscale scores were included as predictors in the same path model. In order to eliminate this multicollinearity, separate path models were estimated for BSI Total scores and BSI subscale scores. No indices of multicollinearity were subsequently observed in either path model (i.e., VIF statistics for all BSI subscale scores were less than 10).

Emotional Abuse and Emotional Neglect Results: Overall Sample

All analyses were conducted in two steps: (a) direct models, indicated by τ in Figure 1, were analyzed to assess the relationship between emotional abuse or emotional neglect and Quality of Marriage Index scores, (b) mediation models, indicated by α, β, and τ` in Figure 1, were analyzed to assess the relationship between emotional abuse or emotional neglect and marital satisfaction scores in the presence of Brief Symptom Inventory total and subscale scores as mediators. All mediation paths were tested for significance using both MacKinnon, Lockwood, and

Hoffman's (1998) distribution of products ($z_\alpha z_\beta$) and distribution of $\alpha\beta/\sigma\alpha\beta$ statistical tests (see MacKinnon, Lockwood, Hoffman, West, & Sheets, 2002).

As shown in Table 4, direct model analysis results indicated a significant negative relationship between both emotional abuse and emotional neglect and Quality of Marriage Index scores; increases in reports of emotional abuse and emotional neglect related significantly to decreases in QMI scores. However, this significant direct effect was no longer statistically significant in the presence of Brief Symptom Inventory total scores, and BSI hostility and depression subscale scores as mediator variables. Increases in emotional abuse and emotional neglect scores were significantly positively related to total scores and hostility and depression subscale scores on the BSI; increases in reported emotional abuse or emotional neglect were related to significant increases in BSI total scores and BSI hostility and depression subscale scores. Significant increases in BSI total scores and BSI hostility and depression subscale scores, in turn, were significantly negatively related to QMI scores; increases in BSI total scores and BSI hostility and depression subscale scores were related to significant decreases in marital satisfaction scores. Following the analyses for the overall sample, separate analyses were performed to examine if the significant mediation results observed for the overall sample were moderated by gender.

Moderated Mediation Results

Emotional abuse and neglect: males. As shown in Table 5, direct model results indicated a significant negative relationship between emotional abuse and marital satisfaction scores for males consistent with results for the overall sample. This significant direct effect was no longer significant in the presence of Brief Symptom Inventory total scores and BSI paranoia subscale scores as moderator variables. Increases in emotional abuse scores were significantly positively related to BSI total scores and paranoia subscale scores. Increases in emotional abuse scores were related to significant increases in BSI total scores and paranoia subscale scores. Increases in BSI total scores and paranoia subscale scores, in turn, were significantly negatively related to marital satisfaction scores; increases in BSI total scores and paranoia subscale scores were related to significant decreases in marital satisfaction. Results of analyses involving emotional neglect showed a

TABLE 4. Overall Results of Mediation Analyses

	b	*S.E.*	*Wald*	β
Emotional Abuse				
Direct Effect				
Emotional Abuse→QMI	−0.35	0.10	−3.64**	−0.31
Mediation: BSI Total				
Emotional Abuse→BSI Total	3.01	0.39	7.72**	0.56
BSI Total→QMI	−0.10	0.02	−4.88**	−0.45
Emotional Abuse→QMI	−0.06	0.11	−0.57	−0.05
Mediation: BSI Hostility and Depression				
Emotional Abuse→Hostility	0.16	0.05	3.25**	0.28
Hostility→QMI	−0.49	0.18	−2.71**	−0.26
Emotional Abuse→QMI	−0.07	0.10	−0.69	−0.06
Emotional Abuse→Depression	0.53	0.08	6.96**	0.52
Depression→QMI	−0.38	0.19	−1.99*	−0.35
Emotional Abuse→QMI	−0.07	0.10	−0.69	−0.06
Emotional Neglect				
Direct Effect				
Emotional Neglect→QMI	−0.37	0.13	−2.80**	−0.24
Mediation: BSI Total				
Emotional Neglect→BSI Total	2.11	0.61	3.48**	0.29
BSI Total→QMI	−0.10	0.02	−5.63**	−0.45
Emotional Neglect→QMI	−0.17	0.12	−1.35	−0.11
Mediation: BSI Hostility and Depression				
Emotional Neglect→Hostility	0.14	0.07	1.99**	0.17
Hostility→QMI	−0.48	0.18	−2.68**	−0.26
Emotional Neglect→QMI	−0.11	0.12	−0.93	−0.07
Emotional Neglect→Depression	0.42	0.12	3.64**	0.30
Depression→QMI	−0.37	0.19	−1.96*	−0.33
Emotional Neglect→QMI	−0.11	0.12	−0.93	−0.07

Note: * = $p < .05$; ** = $p < .01$.

TABLE 5. Results of Mediation Analyses by Gender (Moderated Mediation)

Emotional Abuse–Males				
	b	*S.E.*	*Wald*	β
Direct Effect				
Emotional Abuse→QMI	−0.35	0.13	−2.70**	−0.32
Mediation: BSI Total				
Emotional Abuse→BSI Total	2.25	0.63	3.57**	0.41
BSI Total→QMI	−0.08	0.02	−3.42**	−0.41
Emotional Abuse→QMI	−0.17	0.13	−1.29	−0.15
Mediation: BSI Paranoia				
Emotional Abuse→Paranoia	0.35	0.11	3.06**	0.35
Paranoia→QMI	0.39	0.18	−2.19**	−0.32
Emotional Abuse→QMI	−0.14	0.13	−1.07	−0.12

Note: * = $p < .05$; ** = $p < .01$.

non-significant relationship between emotional neglect and Quality of Marriage Index scores, so no further analyses were conducted.

Emotional abuse and neglect: females. As shown in Tables 6 and 7, direct model results indicated significant negative relationships between emotional abuse and emotional neglect and Quality of Marriage Index scores; increases in emotional abuse or emotional neglect were significantly related to decreases in marital satisfaction. These significant direct effects were no longer statistically significant in the presence of Brief Symptom Inventory total scores, and BSI hostility and obsessive-compulsive subscale scores as mediator variables. Increases in emotional abuse and emotional neglect scores were significantly positively related to BSI total scores, and hostility and obsessive-compulsive subscale scores; increases in reported emotional abuse or emotional neglect were related to significant increases in BSI total scores and hostility and obsessive-compulsive subscale scores. Significant increases in both BSI total scores and hostility and obsessive-compulsive subscale scores were, in turn, significantly related to QMI scores. Specifically, significant increases in BSI total scores and hostility subscale scores were related to significant decreases in marital satisfaction scores, and significant increases in obsessive-compulsive subscale scores were related to significant increases in marital satisfaction scores.

TABLE 6. Results of Mediation Analyses by Gender (Moderated Mediation)

Emotional Abuse–Females				
	b	*S.E.*	*Wald*	β
Direct Effect				
Emotional Abuse→QMI	−0.41	0.14	−2.84**	−0.33
Mediation: BSI Total				
Emotional Abuse→BSI Total	3.70	0.50	7.44**	0.68
BSI Total→QMI	−0.11	0.03	−3.24**	−0.48
Emotional Abuse→QMI	−0.01	0.18	−0.05	−0.01
Mediation: BSI Hostility and Obsession				
Emotional Abuse→Hostility	0.19	0.07	2.60**	0.31
Hostility→QMI	−0.71	0.29	−2.47**	−0.36
Emotional Abuse→QMI	−0.10	0.16	−0.62	−0.08
Emotional Abuse→Obsession	0.55	0.09	5.80**	0.58
Obsession→QMI	0.43	0.20	2.17*	0.33
Emotional Abuse→QMI	−0.10	0.16	−0.62	−0.08

Note: * = $p < .05$; ** = $p < .01$.

TABLE 7. Results of Mediation Analyses by Gender (Moderated Mediation)

Emotional Neglect–Females				
	b	*S.E.*	*Wald*	β
Direct Effect				
Emotional Neglect→QMI	−0.62	0.22	−2.85**	−0.33
Mediation: BSI Total				
Emotional Neglect→BSI Total	3.60	0.93	3.88**	0.43
BSI Total→QMI	−0.09	0.03	−3.51**	−0.42
Emotional Neglect→QMI	−0.28	0.22	−1.27	−0.15
Mediation: BSI Hostility and Obsession				
Emotional Neglect→Hostility	0.37	0.11	3.37**	0.39
Hostility→QMI	−0.67	0.29	−2.30*	−0.34
Emotional Neglect→QMI	−0.07	0.21	−0.32	−0.03
Emotional Neglect→Obsession	0.47	0.17	2.79**	0.33
Obsession→QMI	0.41	0.20	2.09*	0.31
Emotional Neglect→QMI	−0.10	0.16	−0.62	−0.08

Note: * = $p < .05$; ** = $p < .01$.

DISCUSSION

Consistent with past research (e.g., Johnson & Bradbury, 1999), newlywed couples in this study tended to endorse high rates of marital satisfaction on the Quality of Marriage Index. At the same time, a significant minority of newlywed spouses reported experiencing notable psychological distress, as indicated by elevated scores on the Brief Symptom Inventory. High rates of psychological maltreatment also emerged, with 46.7% of participants endorsing emotional abuse and 74.1% reporting emotional neglect. The high rate of emotional *neglect*, in particular, exceeds percentages reported in most community-based investigations. One possible explanation is that all emotional neglect items on the Childhood Trauma Questionnaire, such as "I felt loved," are reversed scored. As a consequence, it is unclear whether the absence of positive endorsement of these items is indeed reflective of participants actual experiences of emotional neglect. Rather, it may be that the items on this scale capture negative, yet sub-threshold parent-child interactions, or tap into a slightly different construct (e.g., family cohesiveness) than emotional neglect per se. Despite this possibility, the victimization rates found here are not entirely unprecedented in the literature. For example, Vissing et al. (1991) reported that 63% of parents admitted using psychologically abusive tactics at least once in the preceding year, while approximately 21% reported repeated use of such tactics (>20 times). Additionally, just as previous research has documented linkages between psychological maltreatment long-term mental health and interpersonal correlates (e.g., Mullen et al., 1996; see review by Twaite & Rodriguez-Srednicki, 2004), results of the current study revealed greater psychological distress and marital dissatisfaction among those reporting heightened levels of psychological maltreatment during childhood. Also mirroring past research (e.g., Davila & Bradbury, 1998; Fruzzetti, 1996; Whisman et al., 2004), significant linkages emerged between adults' psychological symptomatology on every BSI subscale (e.g., depression, somatization, obsessive-compulsive) and self-reported marital dissatisfaction.

Although these results are consistent with past findings, the major goal of the present study was to go beyond examination of individual linkages in order to explore psychological distress as a potential mechanism by which childhood emotional abuse and emotional neglect may impact adult marital satisfaction. As predicted, associations between psychological maltreatment and marital quality in the overall sample were greatly reduced after taking into account various mental health symptoms, specifically overall psychological distress, depression, and hostility. Highlighting the salience of psychological maltreatment, the hypothesized mediational model was supported even when controlling for all other abuse types (child sexual abuse, physical abuse, and physical neglect). These results replicate and extend prior findings with college students (DiLillo et al., in press) and reveal that the impact of psychological maltreatment on later marital satisfaction may operate indirectly via adulthood mental health symptomatology. Of course, mental health functioning may be only one of several pathways by which child psychological maltreatment impinges on the quality of later romantic relationships. For instance, attachment-related processes (e.g., internal working models) also may be an important mechanism (Berlin & Dodge, 2004), particularly in light of recent findings showing that maternal attachment mediates the long-term interpersonal sequelae of child sexual abuse (Liang, Williams, & Siegel, 2006). Although it is likely that other mechanisms such as attachment help explain these relationships, psychological distress appears to be a robust factor–beyond other maltreatment types–in accounting for long-term impacts of psychological maltreatment on marital satisfaction.

Although the mediational analyses were significant for the overall sample, gender was found to moderate these results, revealing slightly different patterns of findings for men and women. Whereas results for the broader sample implicated global psychological distress, hostility, and depression as mediators, the relationship between emotional abuse and marital quality for men was better accounted for by psychological distress and paranoia, while mediational analyses for emotional neglect were not supported. For women, elevated psychological distress, hostility, and obsessive-compulsive scores mediated associations between both psychological abuse and neglect and long-term relational satisfaction or distress.

These gender differences suggest that boys may encounter different forms, levels, or types of psychological maltreatment than do girls, which may subsequently engender different developmental pathways for men and women (Claussen & Crittenden, 1991; DiLillo et al., in press). Specifically, men's elevated paranoia scores, a subscale that inquires about beliefs or feelings that others cannot be trusted or are to blame for one's difficulties, indicate that husbands' marital satisfaction is adversely impacted by suspicious and guarded thoughts. It is possible that men who experienced elevated levels of psychological abuse during childhood, such as being called names or sworn at by caregivers, are less trusting of others' intentions and may carry this distrust and guardedness forward into relations with romantic partners. Another finding that emerged for men was the non-significant relationship between emotional neglect and marital quality. In this study, husbands' and wives reported similar levels of emotional neglect during childhood, yet for men these experiences were not associated with their marital satisfaction. It is possible that husbands' current dyadic satisfaction is simply less sensitive to the influence of the acts of omission that comprise emotional neglect (e.g., feeling loved or emotionally close to parents/caregivers) than to acts of commission (e.g., being called names).

Conversely, with the exception of broad psychological distress, wives appear to experience manifestations of early psychological maltreatment that are distinct from those of husbands. Our finding that hostility was a significant mediator was consistent with past research (DiLillo, Tremblay, & Peterson, 2000), and indicates that feelings of irritation, temper outbursts, frequent arguments, and anger may account for marital quality among women who experienced psychological maltreatment. The finding that increased obsessive-compulsive tendencies, including checking behaviors and difficulties with decision-making, were related to *greater* marital quality was unexpected, especially in light of previous findings linking marital dissatisfaction to obsessive-compulsive disorder (e.g., Riggs, Hiss, & Foa, 1992). However, as Davila and Bradbury (1998) noted, relatively little work has been done to examine the connection between obsessive-compulsive symptomatology and marital quality, suggesting that future research is warranted in order to clarify this relationship.

The present findings replicate and extend previous knowledge about the long-term interpersonal sequelae of psychological maltreatment. However, there are several notable methodological limitations. First, given that the study design is cross-sectional rather than longitudinal, causal conclusions cannot be drawn from these results. Relatedly, the present model assumes that psychological distress precedes relationship dysfunction, even though these constructs were assessed concurrently. Although the statistical robustness of these associations gives credence to our interpretation that psychological maltreatment impacts marital satisfaction through adult mental health symptoms, it is quite possible that mental health functioning is influenced by the quality and satisfaction of the marital relationship. Some research, for instance, has shown that, for women, the relationship between depressive symptomatology and marital dysfunction is cyclical, with depression predicting dyadic distress, which similarly predicts depression (Davila et al., 1997). Although not inclusive of child maltreatment history, longitudinal data have demonstrated differential trajectories for men and women, showing depression leading to marital dissatisfaction for men, with the causal arrow being in the opposite direction for women (Fincham et al., 1997).

A related limitation is the retrospective, self-report nature of the assessments; it is possible that some participants underreported current negative experiences, such as adulthood psychological or marital distress. In addition, although this study used a randomly recruited sample of newlyweds and generated a response rate consistent with other studies using a similar methodology (e.g., Davila et al., 1997), it would be useful for these findings to be replicated with a more ethnically diverse sample. Finally, because couples with children often report increased marital dissatisfaction (Bradbury, Fincham, & Beach, 2000; Clulow, 1991; Twenge, Campbell, & Foster, 2003), future research should aim to understand the role of children in potentially influencing the relationships found here.

Despite limitations, results of this study have the potential to inform clinical interventions for adult survivors of child maltreatment. Given the high prevalence of child abuse in the general population, a number of people seeking treatment for both individual and couples therapy will present with a history of psychological abuse or neglect. For individual clients, there may be clinical utility in thoroughly assessing maltreatment history as well as possible dyadic distress in order to facilitate change at both the individual and couple levels. Moreover, the current findings illuminate the importance of considering the ways in which psychological distress stemming from early abuse may engender marital discord, including dissatisfaction and distress (Leonard, Follette, & Compton, 2006). According to Leonard et al. (2006), "recovery from trauma is more of a journey than a destination, and as such, it is likely that both individual and couple treatment will occur on many trauma survivors' journeys" (p. 382). These results, too, underscore the possibility that the long-term effects of psychological maltreatment may manifest in distinct ways for men and women. Future investigations, employing a longitudinal methodology examining mental health and marital symptoms across several time points, are needed to shed light on the causal and directional processes that underlie long-term individual and dyadic functioning.

REFERENCES

Barnett, O. W., Miller-Perrin, C. L., & Perrin, R. D. (1997). *Family violence across the lifespan: An introduction*. Thousand Oaks, CA: Sage.

Berlin, L. J., & Dodge, K. A. (2004). Relations among relationships. *Child Abuse and Neglect, 28*, 1127-1132.

Bernstein, D. P., & Fink, L. (1998). *Childhood Trauma Questionnaire: A retrospective self-report manual.* San Antonio, TX: The Psychological Corporation.

Bolger, K. E., & Patterson, C. J. (2001). Developmental pathways from child maltreatment to peer rejection. *Child Development, 72,* 549- 568.

Boulet, J., & Boss, M. W. (1991). Reliability and validity of the Brief Symptom Inventory. *Psychological Assessment, 3,* 433-437.

Bradbury, T. N., Fincham, F. D., & Beach, S. R. H. (2000). Research on the nature and determinants of marital satisfaction: A decade in review. *Journal of Marriage and the Family, 62,* 964-980.

Briere, J., & Runtz, M. (1988). Multivariate correlates of childhood psychological and physical maltreatment among university women. *Child Abuse and Neglect, 12,* 331-341.

Briere, J., & Runtz, M. (1990). Differential adult symptomatology associated with three types of child abuse histories. *Child Abuse and Neglect, 14,* 357-364.

Claussen, A. H., & Crittenden, P. M. (1991). Physical and psychological maltreatment: Relations among types of maltreatment. *Child Abuse and Neglect, 15,* 5-18.

Clulow, C. (1991). Partners becoming parents: A question of difference. *Infant Mental Health Journal, 12,* 256-266.

Collins, N. L., Guichard, A. C., Ford, M. B., & Feeney, B. C. (2004). Working models of attachment: New developments and emerging themes. In W. S. Rholes & J. A. Simpson (Eds.), *Adult attachment: Theory, research, and clinical implications* (pp. 196-239). New York, NY: Guilford Press.

Colman, R. A., & Widom, C. S. (2004). Childhood abuse and neglect and adult intimate relationships: A prospective study. *Child Abuse and Neglect, 28,* 1133-1151.

Culp, L. N., & Beach, S. R. H. (1998). Marriage and depressive symptoms: The role and bases of self-esteem differ by gender. *Psychology of Women Quarterly, 22,* 647-663.

Davila, J., & Bradbury, T. N. (1998). Psychopathology and the marital dyad. In L. L. Abate (Ed.), *Family psychopathology: The relational roots of dysfunctional behavior* (pp. 127-157). New York, NY: Guilford Press.

Davila, J., Bradbury, T. N., Cohan, C. L., & Tochluk, S. (1997). Marital functioning and depressive symptoms: Evidence for a stress generation model. *Journal of Personality and Social Psychology, 73,* 849-861.

Davis, J. L., Petretic-Jackson, P. A., & Ting, L. (2001). Intimacy dysfunction and trauma symptomatology: Long-term correlates of different types of child abuse. *Journal of Traumatic Stress, 14,* 63-79.

Derogatis, L. R. (1993). *Brief Symptom Inventory: Administration, scoring, and procedures manual–II.* Minneapolis, MN: National Computer Systems.

Derogatis, L. R. (1994). *Symptom Checklist-90-R: Administration, scoring, and procedures manual–III.* Minneapolis, MN: National Computer Systems.

Derogatis, L. R., & Melisaratos, N. (1983). The Brief Symptom Inventory: An introductory report. *Psychological Medicine, 13,* 595-605.

DiLillo, D., Lewis, T. & DiLoreto-Colgan, A. (in press). Child maltreatment history and subsequent romantic relationships: Exploring a psychological route to dyadic difficulties. *Journal of Aggression, Maltreatment & Trauma.*

DiLillo, D. (2006). [The long-term psychological and interpersonal sequelae of child maltreatment in newlywed couples]. Unpublished raw data.

DiLillo, D., & Long, P. J. (1999). Perceptions of couple functioning among female survivors of child sexual abuse. *Journal of Child Sexual Abuse, 7*, 59-76.
DiLillo, D., Tremblay, G. C., & Peterson, L. (2000). Linking childhood sexual abuse and abusive parenting: The mediating role of maternal anger. *Child Abuse and Neglect, 24*, 767-779.
Du Rocher Schudlich, T. D., Papp, L. M., & Cummings, E. M. (2004). Relations of husbands' and wives' dysphoria to marital conflict resolution strategies. *Journal of Family Psychology, 18*, 171-183.
Edwards, V. J., Holden, G. W., Felitti, V. J., & Anda, R. F. (2003). Relationship between multiple forms of childhood maltreatment and adult mental health in community respondents: Results from the adverse childhood experiences study. *American Journal of Psychiatry, 160*, 1453-1460.
Egeland, B. (1991). A longitudinal study of high-risk families: Issues and findings. In R. H. Starr, Jr., & D. A. Wolfe (Eds.), *The effects of child abuse and neglect: Issues and research* (pp. 33-56). New York, NY: Guilford Press.
Fincham, F. D., Beach, S. R. H., Harold, G. T., & Osborne, L. N. (1997). Marital satisfaction and depression: Different causal relationships for men and women? *Psychological Science, 8*, 351-357.
Fortin, A., & Chamberland, C. (1995). Preventing the psychological maltreatment of children. *Journal of Interpersonal Violence, 10*, 275-295.
Fruzzetti, A. E. (1996). Causes and consequences: Individual distress in the context of couple interactions. *Journal of Consulting and Clinical Psychology, 64*, 1192-1201.
Gibb, B. E. (2002). Childhood maltreatment and negative cognitive styles: A quantitative and qualitative review. *Clinical Psychology Review, 22*, 223-246.
Gibb, B. E., Alloy, L. B., Abramson, L. Y., & Marx, B. P. (2003). Childhood maltreatment and maltreatment-specific inferences: A test of Rose and Abramson's (1992) extension of the hopelessness theory. *Cognition and Emotion, 17*, 917-931.
Gibb, B. E., Alloy, L. B., Abramson, L. Y., Rose, D. T., Whitehouse, W. G., & Hogan, M. E. (2001). Childhood maltreatment and college students' current suicidal ideation: A test of the hopelessness theory. *Suicide and Life-Threatening Behavior, 31*, 405-415.
Glaser, D. (2002). Emotional abuse and neglect (psychological maltreatment): A conceptual framework. *Child Abuse and Neglect, 26*, 697-714.
Hair, J. F., Anderson, R. E., Tatham, R. L., & Black, W. (1998). *Multivariate data analysis* (5th ed.). Upper Saddle River, NJ: Prentice Hall.
Halford, W. K., Sanders, M. R., & Behrens, B. C. (2000). Repeating the errors of our parents? Family-of-origin spouse violence and observed conflict management in engaged couples. *Family Process, 39*, 219-235.
Hart, S. N., & Brassard, M. R. (1987). A major threat to children's mental health: Psychological maltreatment. *American Psychologist, 42*, 160-165.
Hart, S. N., Brassard, M. R., & Karlson, H. C. (1996). Psychological maltreatment. In J. Briere, L. Berliner, J. A. Bulkley, C. Jenny, & T. Reid (Eds.), *The APSAC handbook on child maltreatment* (pp. 72-89). Thousand Oaks, CA: Sage.
Hart, S. N., Brassard, M. R., Binggeli, N. J., & Davidson, H. A. (2002). Psychological maltreatment. In J. E. B. Myers, L. Berliner, J. Briere, C. T. Hendrix, C. Jenny, & T. A. Reid (Eds.), *The APSAC handbook on child maltreatment* (2nd ed., pp. 79-103). Thousand Oaks, CA: Sage.

Hayes, J. A. (1997). What does the Brief Symptom Inventory measure in college and university counseling center clients? *Journal of Counseling Psychology, 44*, 360-367.

Heyman, R. E., Sayers, S. L., & Bellack, A. S. (1994). Global marital satisfaction versus marital adjustment: An empirical comparison of three measures. *Journal of Family Psychology, 8*, 432-446.

Johnson, M. D., & Bradbury, T. N. (1999). Marital satisfaction and topographical assessment of marital interaction: A longitudinal analysis of newlywed couples. *Personal Relationships, 6*, 19-40.

Kairys, S. W., Johnson, C. F., & the Committee on Child Abuse and Neglect (2002). The psychological maltreatment of children–Technical report. *Pediatrics, 109*. Retrieved August 20, 2006, from http://www.pediatrics.org/cgi/content/full/109/4/e68

Karney, B. R., Davila, J., Cohan, C. L., Sullivan, K. T., Johnson, M. D., & Bradbury, T. N. (1995). An empirical investigation of sampling strategies in marital research. *Journal of Marriage and the Family, 57*, 909-920.

Kline, R. B. (2005). *Principles and practice of structural equation modeling* (2nd ed.). New York, NY: Guilford Press.

Krause, E. D., Mendelson, T., & Lynch, T. R. (2003). Childhood emotional invalidation and adult psychological distress: The mediating role of emotional inhibition. *Child Abuse and Neglect, 27*, 199-213.

Kurdek, L. A. (1995). Predicting change in marital satisfaction from husbands' and wives' conflict resolution styles. *Journal of Marriage and the Family, 57*, 153-164.

Kurdek, L. A. (2002). Predicting the timing of separation and marital satisfaction: An eight-year prospective longitudinal study. *Journal of Marriage and the Family, 64*, 163-179.

Kurdek, L. A. (2005). Gender and marital satisfaction early in marriage: A growth curve approach. *Journal of Marriage and the Family, 67*, 68-84.

Leonard, L. M., Follette, V. M., & Compton, J. S. (2006). A principle-based intervention for couples affected by trauma. In V. M. Follette & J. I. Ruzek (Eds.), *Cognitive-behavioral therapies for trauma* (pp. 362-387). New York, NY: Guilford Press.

Liang, B., Williams, L. M., & Siegel, J. A. (2006). Relational outcomes of childhood sexual trauma in female survivors: A longitudinal study. *Journal of Interpersonal Violence, 21*, 42-57.

Loos, M. E., & Alexander, P. C. (1997). Differential effects associated with self-reported histories of abuse and neglect in a college sample. *Journal of Interpersonal Violence, 12*, 340-360.

MacKinnon, D. P., Lockwood, C., & Hoffman, J. (1998, June). *A new method to test for mediation*. Paper presented at the annual meeting of the Society for Prevention research, Park City, UT.

MacKinnon, D. P., Lockwood, C. M., Hoffman, J. M., West, S. G., & Sheets, V. (2002). A comparison of methods to test mediation and other intervening variable effects. *Psychological Methods, 7*, 83-104.

Medrano, M. A., Zule, W. A., Hatch, J., & Desmond, D. P. (1999). Prevalence of childhood trauma in a community sample of substance-abusing women. *American Journal of Drug and Alcohol Abuse, 25*, 449-462.

Moeller, T. P., Bachmann, G. A., & Moeller, J. R. (1993). The combined effects of physical, sexual, and emotional abuse during childhood: Long-term health consequences for women. *Child Abuse and Neglect, 17*, 623-640.
Moran, P. B., Vuchinich, S., & Hall, N. K. (2004). Associations between types of maltreatment and substance use during adolescence. *Child Abuse and Neglect, 28*, 565-574.
Mullen, P. E., Martin, J. L., Anderson, J. C., Romans, S. E., & Herbison, G. P. (1996). The long-term impact of the physical, emotional, and sexual abuse of children: A community study. *Child Abuse and Neglect, 20*, 7-21.
Norton, R. (1983). Measuring marital quality: A critical look at the dependent variable. *Journal of Marriage and the Family, 45*, 141-151.
O'Hagan, K. P. (1995). Emotional and psychological abuse: Problems of definition. *Child Abuse and Neglect, 19*, 449-461.
Paivio, S. C., & Cramer, K. M. (2004). Factor structure and reliability of the Childhood Trauma Questionnaire in a Canadian undergraduate student sample. *Child Abuse and Neglect, 28*, 889-904.
Prince, S. E., & Jacobson, N. S. (1995). A review and evaluation of marital and family therapies for affective disorders. *Journal of Marital and Family Therapy, 21*, 377-401.
Riggs, D. S., Hiss, H., & Foa, E. B. (1992). Marital distress and the treatment of obsessive compulsive disorder. *Behavior Therapy, 23*, 585-597.
Rodgers, C. S., Lang, A. J., Laffaye, C., Satz, L. E., Dresselhaus, T. R., & Stein, M. B. (2004). The impact of individual forms of childhood maltreatment on health behavior. *Child Abuse and Neglect, 28*, 575-586.
Rogge, R. D., & Bradbury, T. N. (1999). Till violence does us part: The differing roles of communication and aggression in predicting adverse marital outcomes. *Journal of Consulting and Clinical Psychology, 67*, 340-351.
Scher, C. D., Forde, D. R., McQuaid, J. R., & Stein, M. B. (2004). Prevalence and demographic correlates of childhood maltreatment in an adult community sample. *Child Abuse and Neglect, 28*, 167-180.
Scher, C. D., Stein, M. B., Asmundson, G. J. G., McCreary, D. R., & Forde, D. R. (2001). The Childhood Trauma Questionnaire in a community sample: Psychometric properties and normative data. *Journal of Traumatic Stress, 14*, 843-857.
Spertus, I. L., Yehuda, R., Wong, C. M., Halligan, S., & Seremetis, S. V. (2003). Childhood emotional abuse and neglect as predictors of psychological and physical symptoms in women presenting to a primary care practice. *Child Abuse and Neglect, 27*, 1247-1258.
Stevens, J. P. (2002). *Applied multivariate statistics for the social sciences* (4th ed.). Mahwah, NJ: Lawrence Erlbaum Associates.
Straus, M. A., & Field, C. J. (2003). Psychological aggression by American parents: National data on prevalence, chronicity, and severity. *Journal of Marriage and the Family, 65*, 795-808.
Thomas, P. M. (2003). Protection, dissociation, and internal roles: Modeling and treating the effects of child abuse. *Review of General Psychology, 7*, 364-380.
Thompson, R. A., Laible, D. J., & Ontai, L. L. (2003). Early understandings of emotion, morality, and self: Developing a working model. *Advances in Child Development and Behavior, 31*, 137-171.

Twaite, J. A., & Rodriguez-Srednicki, O. (2004). Understanding and reporting child abuse: Legal and psychological perspectives: Part two: Emotional abuse and secondary abuse. *The Journal of Psychiatry and Law, 32*, 443-481.

Twenge, J. M., Campbell, W. K., & Foster, C. A. (2003). Parenthood and marital satisfaction: A meta-analytic review. *Journal of Marriage and the Family, 65*, 574-583.

Vissing, Y. M., Straus, M. A., Gelles, R. J., & Harrop, J. W. (1991). Verbal aggression by parents and psychosocial problems of children. *Child Abuse and Neglect, 15*, 223-238.

Wark, M. J., Kruczek, T., & Boley, A. (2003). Emotional neglect and family structure: Impact on student functioning. *Child Abuse and Neglect, 27*, 1033-1043.

Whisman, M. A., & Delinsky, S. S. (2002). Marital satisfaction and an information-processing measure of partner-schemas. *Cognitive Therapy and Research, 26*, 617-627.

Whisman, M. A., Uebelacker, L. A., & Weinstock, L. M. (2004). Psychopathology and marital satisfaction: The importance of evaluating both partners. *Journal of Consulting and Clinical Psychology, 72*, 830-838.

doi:10.1300/J135v07n02_07

Index

